Diet & Stress

Simple Solutions

Is what you're eating, eating you?

Vicki Griffin, PhD, MACN
Edwin Neblett, MD, MPH
Evelyn Kissinger, MS, RD, IBCLC

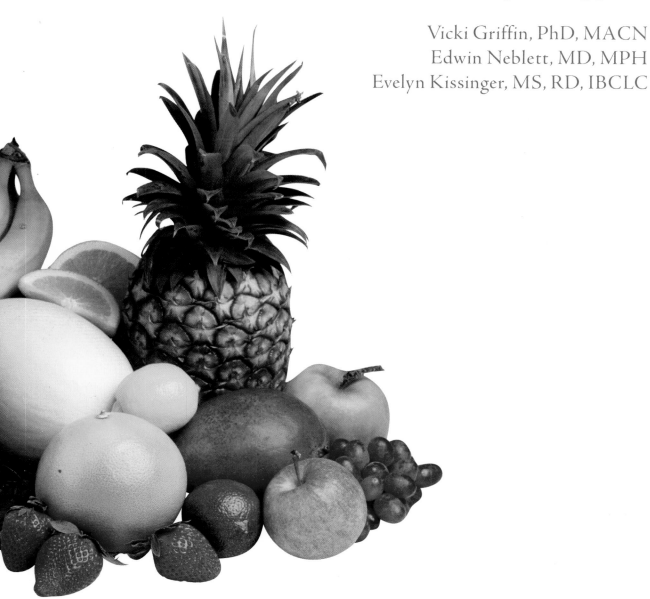

CONTENTS

FOREWORD

Many people think of diet as only affecting their risk for physical problems like obesity, diabetes, elevated cholesterol, high blood pressure, heart disease, and cancer. But dietary intake is not only crucial for the prevention of chronic diseases, it also has an unexpected effect on our daily life. Well-balanced nutrition is essential, not optional, for both mental and physical well-being.

Even when individuals understand that diet profoundly affects mental function and the ability to cope with stress, its importance is often ignored, especially when a person feels overwhelmed by stress from many sources, including zany schedules, unexpected demands, deadlines, financial challenges, sleep deficit, and lack of exercise.

There are several things we want to accomplish for you in this book. First, we take a look at the overall problem of stress in our society and give you an opportunity to assess how you would place yourself in the stress picture.

Second, we examine some of the ways that prolonged or severe stress affects the body's use of nutrients and increases the need for good nutrition.

Well-balanced nutrition is essential, not optional, for both mental and physical well-being.

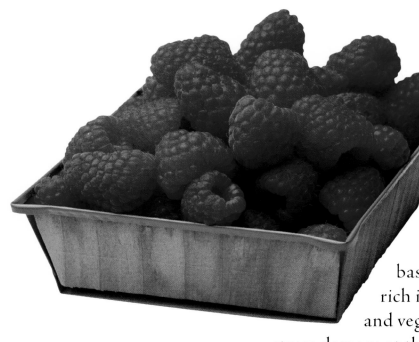

Third, we show how poor nutrition and eating habits actually increase stress-proneness, the intensity of the stress response, and the length of time it takes for stress levels to return to normal.

Fourth, we take a look at plant-based nutrition and examine how a diet rich in whole grains, legumes, fresh fruits and vegetables, nuts and seeds can diminish stress damage at the cellular and hormonal level, and help you to be more resilient under stress both emotionally and physically.

You will also find a number of eye-opening illustrations comparing the calories in a typical fast food meal or certain types of snacks with healthy options.

For example, to get the calories in a typical 2,000-calorie fast food burger meal, you could go to the grocery store and buy about 12 pounds of fresh vegetables! You definitely get more bounce by the ounce with plant nutrition in terms of dollars, nutrition, and stress protection!

We have included a variety of healthy, fast, easy recipes for you to try, and offer other health materials and videos advertised in the back of this book. We want you to have recipes that not only taste good and have lots of stress-protective nutrients, but we know that busy people need food that is fast, easy, economical, versatile, and portable!

For example, to get the calories in a typical 2,000-calorie fast food burger meal, you could go to the grocery store and buy about 12 pounds of fresh vegetables!

You will also find a special section entitled "Lowering stress...one bite at a time." This is designed to help you make simple changes in your daily eating routine that will help build nervous system strength, lower your risk of chronic lifestyle diseases, give you more meal satisfaction, and provide real strength rather than artificial stimulation. One thing is certain: when you eat better, you will feel better. And when you feel better, life is better!

We have also included some simple stress reduction tips that will help you manage the seemingly endless challenges and stressors that can drain you emotionally and physically.

Each section in this book is followed by a personal evaluation sheet that gives you an opportunity to examine some of your personal

When you eat better, you will feel better. And when you feel better, life is better!

habits and explore simple ways to make healthful changes that will work for you. We have included helpful Bible texts that you can look up to find counsel and promises as you adopt new ways of eating and managing stress in your life.

It is our heartfelt prayer that the information in this book will help you take personal steps toward better physical and mental health and provide you with some simple tools for boosting your ability to cope with stress in a stressful world!

~The Authors

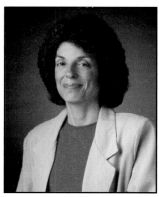
Vicki Griffin

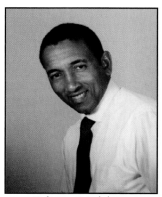
Edwin Neblett

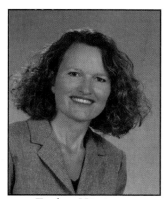
Evelyn Kissinger

Startling
Statistics

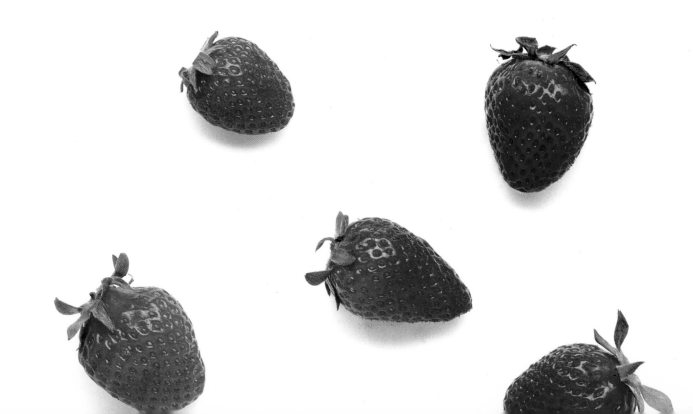

One out of every four, or 26 percent, of adults surveyed said they felt an impending nervous breakdown.

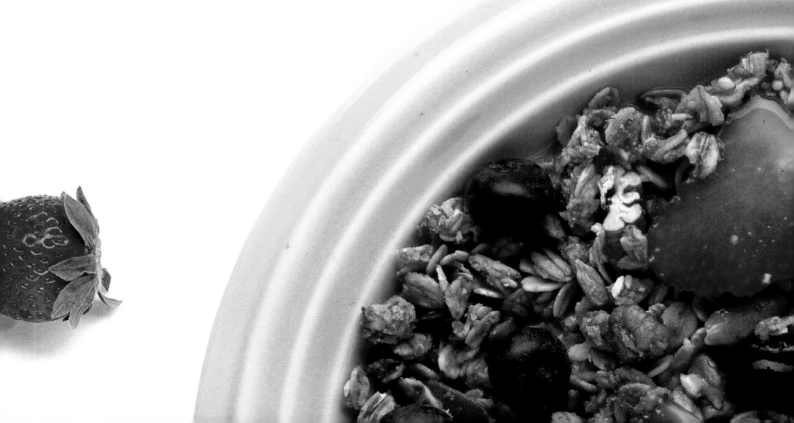

Combine the following in a large bowl and mix well:

8 cups	Quick oats
2 cups	Oat or wheat bran
1 cup	Cornmeal
1 cup	Wheat germ
2 tsp.	Salt
1 cup	Chopped nuts

In a separate container mix together:

¼ cup	Oil (optional)
1 12-oz.	Can unsweetened frozen apple juice
2 T	Molasses
2 tsp.	Vanilla

Stir liquids into dry ingredients, mixing well and breaking up all lumps. Spread out evenly on 2 sprayed cookie sheets or in casserole dishes.

Bake at 250 degrees for 75-90 minutes, stirring every 15-20 minutes to ensure even drying. If cereal starts browning too quickly, reduce oven temperature and finish cooking time.

Turn off heat and allow cereal to **remain in the oven until cool** to complete the drying process. Store in airtight container in a cool, dry place.

✦ **Makes 13 cups of cereal.**

Serving Suggestions

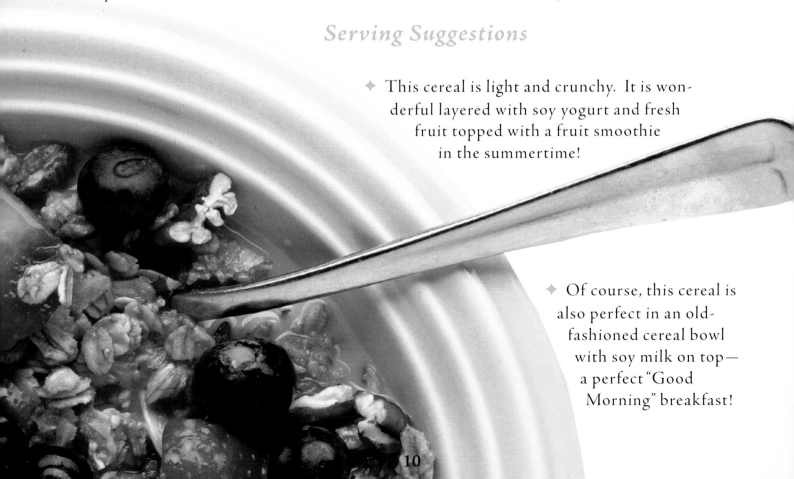

✦ This cereal is light and crunchy. It is wonderful layered with soy yogurt and fresh fruit topped with a fruit smoothie in the summertime!

✦ Of course, this cereal is also perfect in an old-fashioned cereal bowl with soy milk on top— a perfect "Good Morning" breakfast!

"If misery loves company, then misery has company enough."
~Henry Thoreau

I saw her on the refrigerator of an overworked, overweight oncology nurse. No, she wasn't a real person. "She" was a caricature of a highly agitated woman, complete with eyes bulging and hair on end. The caption beneath perfectly described her condition—and the state of many Americans today: "I have one nerve left, and you are about to get on it!"

Stress—it's a part of life. According to a survey conducted by Princeton Survey Research Associates, two-thirds of Americans report being "stressed-out" at least once a week. In 1996, one out of every four, or 26 percent, of adults surveyed said they felt an impending nervous breakdown.[1]

Americans today are plagued with chronic tension, fatigue, anxiety, and stress-related diseases, and many seem powerless to stop their self-destructive course. Experts estimate that almost 20 million people in the United States suffer from chronic depression at an annual cost of 47.3 billion dollars.[2] That figure includes not only direct costs but also the cost associated with 200 million days lost from work each year, at a price tag of about $600 per depressed worker.[3] About 30,000 Americans

"Depression ranks among the top three workplace problems for employee assistance professionals, following only family crisis and stress."

Employee Assistance Professional Association 1996 survey

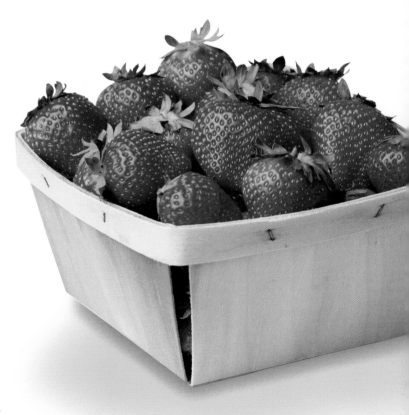

commit suicide each year—that's 1½ times more than the number who are victims of homicide. In addition, approximately 650,000 people in the U.S. attempt to take their lives every year. It is likely that many of these problems are related to chronic stress and depression.

Trickle-Down Stress

Tension and stress are major problems among adults. All this tension is trickling down to the younger set as well. Ronald Kessler, lead researcher in the National Co-morbidity Study of more than 8,000 Americans, reported that among 15- to 24-year-olds, almost one out of every four had serious depression in their teens. Suicide rates for U.S. children and teens increased fourfold between 1950 and 1995, another sign of depression's toll.

Stress is taking its toll on the very youngest Americans, too. In December of 1999, Surgeon General David Satcher released a report showing that 20% of U.S. children suffered from psychiatric

continued on p. 16

Among 15- to 24-year-olds, almost 1 out of every 4 had serious depression in their teens.

The Economic Cost of Depression

- In 1996, 26% of adults felt an impending nervous breakdown[1]

- Antidepressant use up 56% from 1993 (SSRIs)[2]

- 20 million experience clinical depression each year

- 200 million lost work days

- Annual cost: $600 per depressed worker[3]

- 23% of teens suffered serious depression before age 20[4]

- 20% of U.S. children suffer from psychiatric disorders

- Child use of antidepressants up 200% from 1991-95

- Threefold increase of Ritalin use in two- to four-year-olds, Midwestern states[5]

- 30,000 Americans commit suicide every year

- 650,000 people in the United States attempt suicide each year[6]

The High Cost of Stress

The Economic Cost of Depression

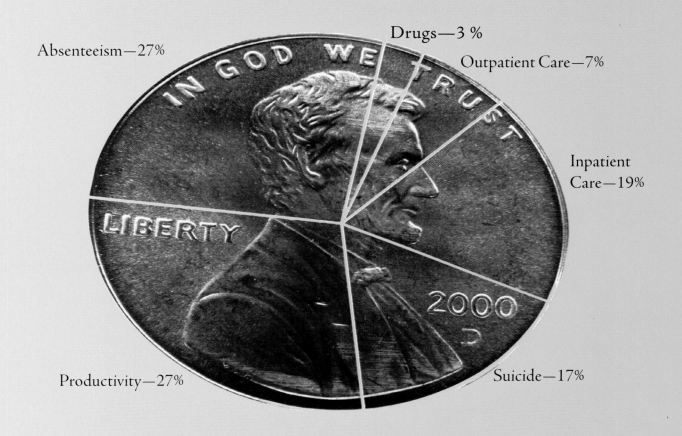

Absenteeism—27%

Drugs—3 %

Outpatient Care—7%

Inpatient Care—19%

Suicide—17%

Productivity—27%

Depression costs 43.2 billion dollars a year

- ✦ 1.2 billion spent on drugs

- ✦ 2.9 billion spent on outpatient care

- ✦ 8.3 billion spent on inpatient care

- ✦ 7.5 billion spent on suicide

- ✦ 12.1 billion: cost of productivity loss

- ✦ 11.2 billion: cost of absenteeism[7]

Reprinted with permission from the *Journal of Clinical Psychology*, 1993;4:425

Social Readjustment

Compute your score on the basis of life events you have experienced in the past two years. Scores predict chance of illness or accident due to stress from changes taking place in your life.[1]

0-150	No significant problems; low stress zone based on life-change criteria (no predictable risk)
150-199	Mild life crisis (33% risk)
200-299	Moderate life crisis (50% risk)
300 +	Major life crisis (80% risk)

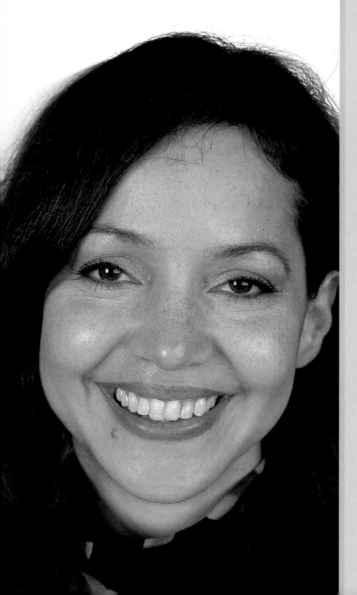

Life Event	Stress Value	
Death of spouse	100	_____
Divorce	73	_____
Marital separation	65	_____
Jail term	63	_____
Death of close family member	63	_____
Personal injury or illness	53	_____
Marriage	50	_____
Fired at work	47	_____
Marital reconciliation	45	_____
Retirement	45	_____
Change in health of family member	44	_____
Pregnancy	40	_____
Sex difficulties	39	_____
Gain of new family member	39	_____
Business adjustment	39	_____
Change in financial state	38	_____
Death of close friend	37	_____
Change to different line of work	36	_____
Change in number of arguments with spouse	35	_____
Mortgage or loan for major purchase (home, etc.)	31	_____
Foreclosure of mortgage or loan	30	_____
Change in responsibilities at work	29	_____
Son or daughter leaving home	29	_____

Rating Scale ✓

Reprinted by permission of the *Journal of Psychosomatic Research*, vol. 11, no. 2. pp. 213–218. Thomas H. Holmes and Richard R. Rahe, "The Social Readjustment Rating Scale," Elsevier Science Inc.

If your score indicates a predictably high risk of illness or accident due to the amount of changes that have occurred in your life in the past two years, consider the following suggestions:

1. Deliberately slow the rate of change taking place in your life in those areas over which you have some control.
2. Take care to eat a healthy diet and get regular exercise that is medically appropriate to your physical ability and level of health.
3. Be especially attentive while driving or working around machinery.
4. Schedule times for relaxation and simple, enjoyable activities on a regular basis.

Life Event	Stress Value	
Trouble with in-laws	29	_____
Outstanding personal achievement	28	_____
Spouse begins or stops work	26	_____
Begin or end school	26	_____
Change in living conditions	25	_____
Revision of personal habits	24	_____
Trouble with boss	23	_____
Change in work hours or conditions	20	_____
Change in residence	20	_____
Change in school	20	_____
Change in recreation	19	_____
Change in church activities	19	_____
Change in social activities	18	_____
Mortgage or loan for lesser purchase (appliances, etc.)	17	_____
Change in sleeping habits	16	_____
Change in number of family get-togethers	15	_____
Change in eating habits	15	_____
Vacation	13	_____
Christmas	12	_____
Minor violations of the law (traffic ticket, etc.)	11	_____
Total		_____

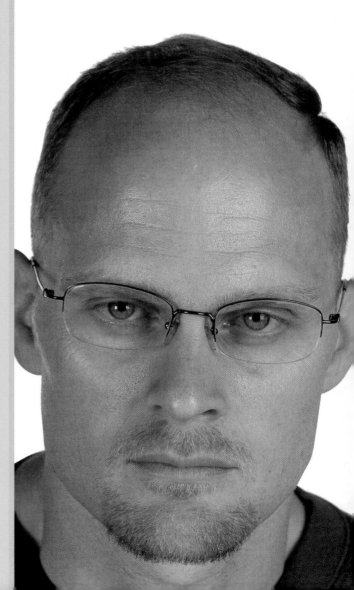

disorders.[4] The number of preschool children on antidepressants jumped more than 200 percent between 1991 and 1995. Ritalin use for two- to four-year-olds during that same time shot up 300 percent in Midwestern states.[5] To be healthy in an increasingly hectic, complex, and fragmented society requires awareness of practical and healthful lifestyle principles. It also requires an unswerving commitment to preserving a sound body, mind, and spirit. Being healthy involves recognizing that all aspects of life are interrelated and need to be balanced if you are to reach your full potential.

Sometimes life seems to be a virtual sea of stress. What impact does stress have on your health? How does it work, and what, if anything, can you do about it? Is it possible to make nutrition and lifestyle choices that will make a difference? Can you choose nutrition and lifestyle options that protect against the ravages of stress, decrease stress-proneness, calms the nerves, and increases your ability to cope when stress does come? Or, can you make nutrition and lifestyle choices that cause even more stress for your body? Although a relatively new field, research is definitely showing that nutrition choices can have a profound effect on the stress response.

In many ways our society has changed. It has become more complex, and in many ways, more demanding. But physiological mechanisms for coping with adversity,

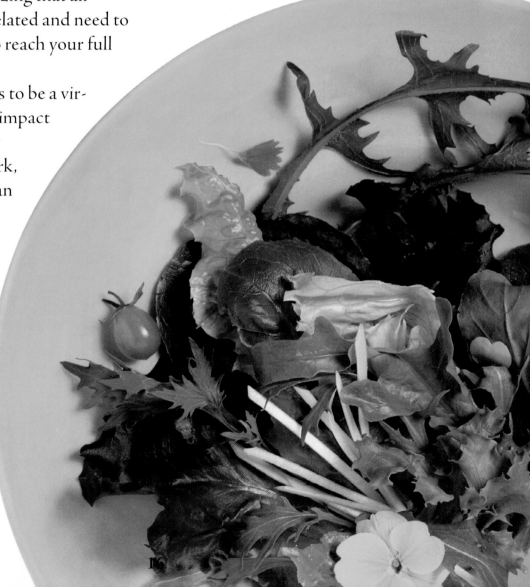

meeting social pressures, information-overload, rapid change, poor nutrition, and even outright threats to survival have not changed! Today, stress is a part of life—and good nutrition is part of the solution.

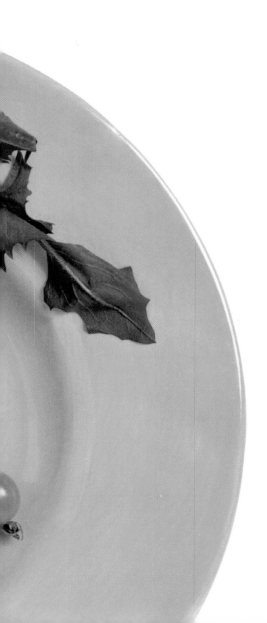

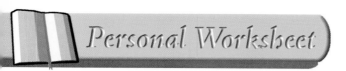

Personal Worksheet

1. Look up Luke 21:25-28. During what time period does the Bible recognize stress as being a special problem?

_____

_____

_____

2. In what ways do I see the problems of stress and tension manifested in society?

_____

_____

_____

3. What specific ways do I find myself caught in a web of stress?

_____

_____

_____

4. Look up 2 Corinthians 4:8-9. What is God's plan for His children during troubled times?

_____

_____

_____

5. Look up Romans 13:12-14. What does it mean to "put on the Lord Jesus?"

_____

_____

_____

6. In what spiritual and practical ways can I minimize the stress trap?

_____

_____

_____

(see answers on page 122)

Metabolic Mishaps

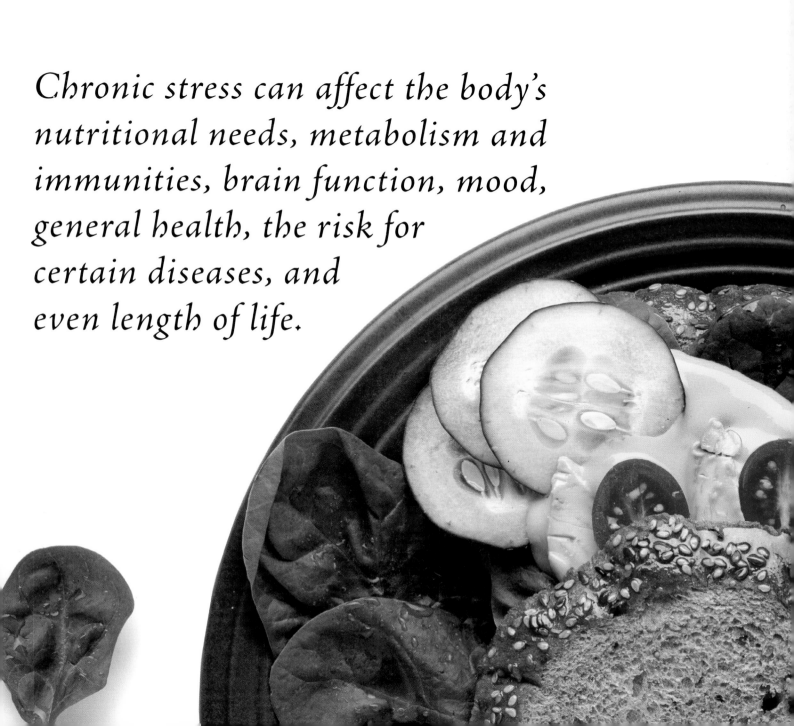

Chronic stress can affect the body's nutritional needs, metabolism and immunities, brain function, mood, general health, the risk for certain diseases, and even length of life.

Mix in blender:

1 cup	Water
¾ cup	Cashews, raw
3 T	Sesame tahini
1 tsp.	Salt
4 T	Nutritional yeast flakes
2 tsp.	Onion powder
½ tsp.	Garlic powder
¼ tsp.	Dill weed
½ cup	Pimiento
4 T	Lemon juice

Pour into sauce pan and thicken over medium heat, stirring constantly.

✦ **Makes 3 cups.**

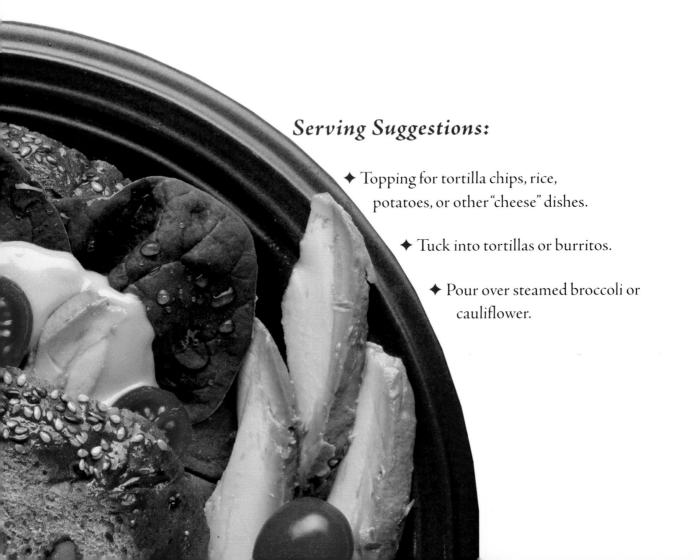

Serving Suggestions:

✦ Topping for tortilla chips, rice, potatoes, or other "cheese" dishes.

✦ Tuck into tortillas or burritos.

✦ Pour over steamed broccoli or cauliflower.

"Can a man take fire in his bosom, and his clothes not be burned?"
~Proverbs 6:27

Not all stress is bad. In fact, some stress adds pleasure, excitement, and energy to various activities. A healthy level of stress-system activity can promote intellectual and emotional growth and sharpen your senses for life's challenges.

But often, stress is not mild and brief but sustained beyond belief! It is this type of prolonged, uncontrollable, emotional, physical, or physiological stress that can cause debility, disease, and even death. But what exactly is stress?

"Stress" is a well-known, often used, but often ill-defined term. It has different meanings for different people. Actually, stress is a term the psychological sciences borrowed from the field of engineering, and it is defined in psychology as "a state of disharmony, dis-equilibrium, or threatened homeostasis."[6] Perhaps a more practical definition would be "the sum total of our responses to the various forces (or stressors) impinging on our lives."[7]

These forces can be physical, emotional, chemical, environmental, spiritual, or symbolic in nature. Simply stated, a stressor is any disturbing factor that disrupts physiological, physical, or mental balance.

Examples of Stressors

PHYSICAL: Can be local (bee sting, laceration, burn) or general (fever, autoimmune disease, diabetes)
EMOTIONAL: Strong emotions, either intrinsic (generated from within) or extrinsic (response to others)
CHEMICAL: Physiologic response to substances such as caffeine, alcohol, high fat, high sugar, etc.
ENVIRONMENTAL: Physiologic responses to external stressors such as noise, pollution, crowding, etc.
SPIRITUAL: Changes that occur in response to feelings of guilty conscience, sense of wrongdoing, etc.
SYMBOLIC: Changes triggered by memories or visual cues that elicit strong emotional response.

(Depending on the length and magnitude of the stressor, and the intensity of the reaction to it, nutritional status and need may be altered.)[1]

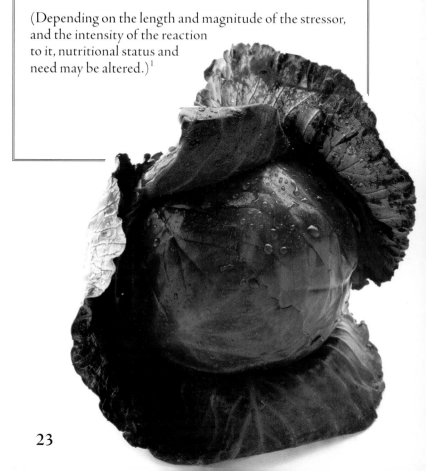

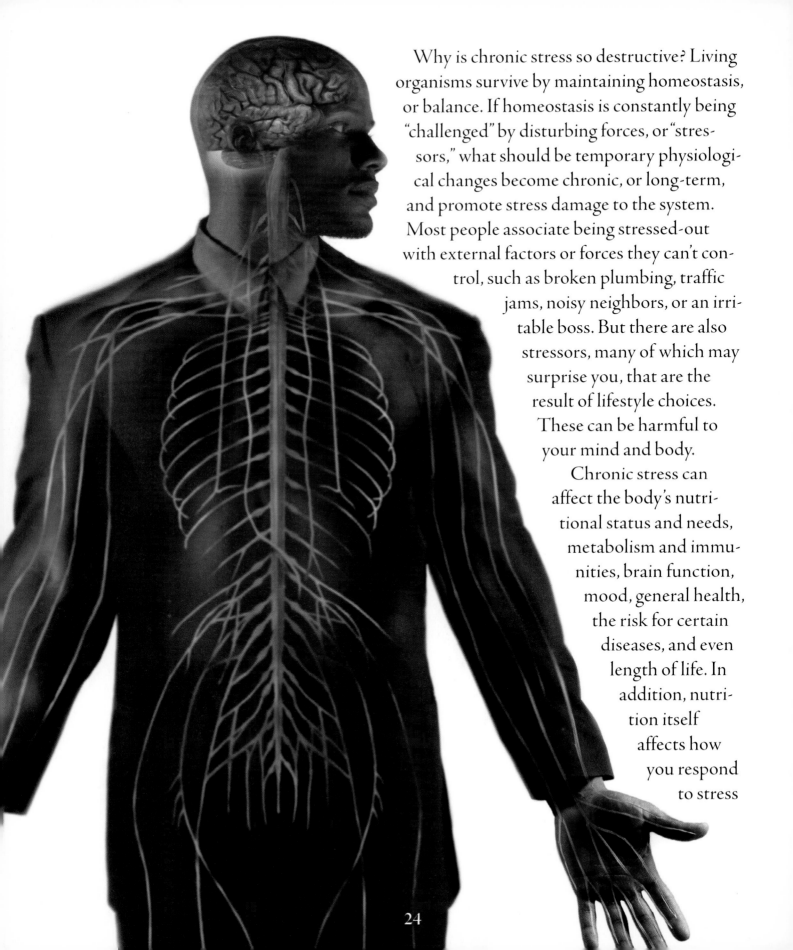

Why is chronic stress so destructive? Living organisms survive by maintaining homeostasis, or balance. If homeostasis is constantly being "challenged" by disturbing forces, or "stressors," what should be temporary physiological changes become chronic, or long-term, and promote stress damage to the system. Most people associate being stressed-out with external factors or forces they can't control, such as broken plumbing, traffic jams, noisy neighbors, or an irritable boss. But there are also stressors, many of which may surprise you, that are the result of lifestyle choices. These can be harmful to your mind and body.

Chronic stress can affect the body's nutritional status and needs, metabolism and immunities, brain function, mood, general health, the risk for certain diseases, and even length of life. In addition, nutrition itself affects how you respond to stress and how much damage the stress response can do!

Prolonged stress also affects people in different ways, depending on the magnitude, length, and timing of the stressful event. Stress is capable of exerting its influence upon the metabolism and function of virtually every system of the body, including the brain, nerves, muscles, organs, glands, and blood vessels. The stress response is greatly varied among individuals, largely depending on your genetic makeup, constitutional strengths and weaknesses, general health, personality type, and environmental factors.[8]

But regardless of all these factors, good nutrition is one of nature's ways of helping every person cope with and fend off the ravages of stress.

Stress Symptoms!

You've most likely experienced common stress symptoms such as a queasy stomach, rapid heartbeat, shallow breathing, dry mouth, headache, and clammy skin. But did you know that stress can also cause mental symptoms such as irritability, forgetfulness, agitation, depression, volatile emotions, fatigue, and confusion? The fact is stress can manifest itself in a large array of symptoms.

Exactly what happens inside your body when stress hits? Your normal stress response is a beneficial, God-given protection. During a stress response, more than a thousand physiochemical reactions take place in your body that enhance awareness, perception, strength, memory, and other defense mechanisms. In the short-term, that's good. But when physical or emotional stress becomes chronic or excessive, physical and mental changes occur that tear down the body's defenses instead of protecting them.[9]

As a result, chronic stress can result in "feelings of fatigue, lack of energy, irritability, demoralization, and hostility."[10] Diseases that are often linked to diet and lifestyle factors, such as insulin resistance, diabetes, heart disease, elevated cholesterol and triglycerides, high blood pressure, osteoporosis, and vascular dementia, are also linked to increased stress-system activity.[11][12][13]

Because your body has been created with a biological priority of survival, it adapts to chronic stress challenges, even at the expense of long-term health. Your body has two major adaptive systems: the neuroendocrine and the immune system. During a stressful situation, they "talk to each other" in a biological attempt to

Chronic stress can result in "feelings of fatigue, lack of energy, irritability, demoralization, and hostility."

25

Physical Effects of Stress

- Queasy stomach
- Shallow breathing
- Nervous perspiration
- Rapid heart beat
- Headache
- Sporadic eating
- Increased hunger
- Loss of appetite

- Clammy skin
- Dry mouth
- PMS or loss of menstruation
- Change in sleep habits
- Lowered immunities
- Muscle pain, spasms
- Substance abuse

Mental Effects of Stress

- Volatile emotions
- Social conflict
- Ambivalence
- Restlessness, tension
- Job absenteeism
- Erratic productivity
- Procrastination
- Perfectionism

- Forgetfulness
- Poor concentration
- Mental sluggishness
- Agitation, anxiety
- Excessive talking
- Irritability
- Depression
- Fatigue

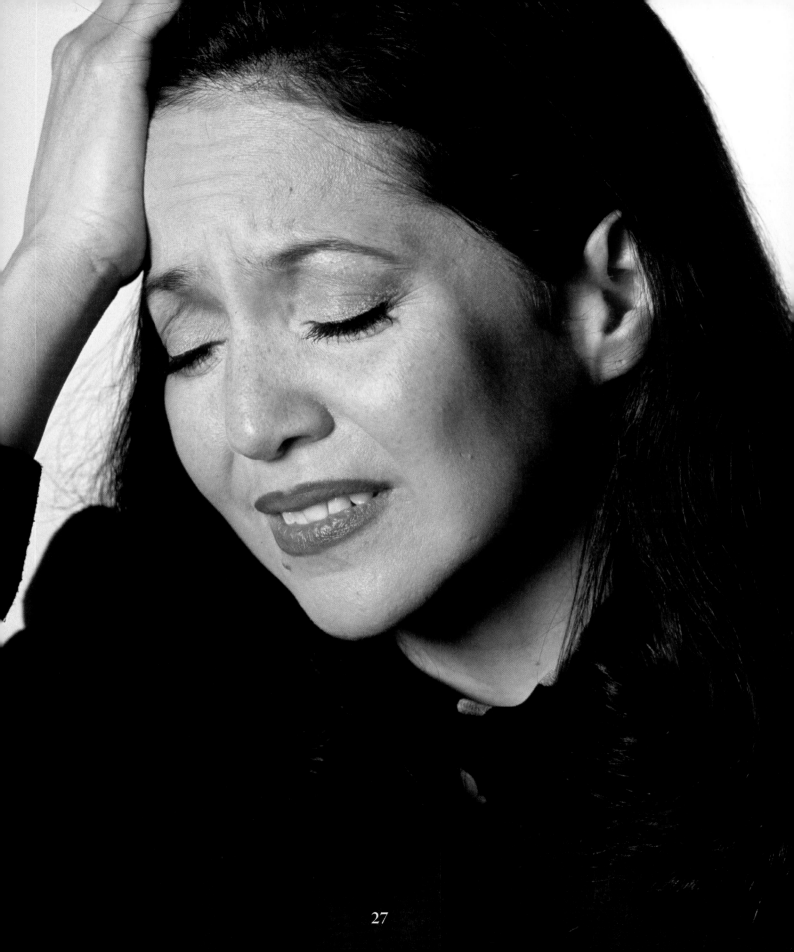

maintain proper balance, or homeostasis.[14]

The two major pathways in this "cross-talk" are the hypothalamic-pituitary-adrenal (**HPA**) axis and the sympathetic nervous system, which produce various stress hormones such as cortisol and adrenaline.[15] These stress hormones in turn affect the muscles, glands, organs, and vessels of the body in various ways.

Repeated stress challenges (which include an unhealthful diet) can eventually

> *"Dysregulation of the stress system … involves a number of human health problems of enormous impact to society."*
>
> *Journal of the American Medical Association,* 1992;267(9):1244-1252

result in either chronic overproduction or underproduction of stress hormones.[16] To understand these two scenarios, think of an abused automobile. In one case (overproduction of stress hormones), the driver has the pedal to the metal, and the result is a high-speed crash with all systems out of control. In the second scenario (underproduction of stress hormones), the driver is cruising along with a burned-out alternator, so the malfunctioning vehicle has only as much push as the battery can pull before it finally fizzles out.

Chronic, or long-term, increase in stress-system activity is associated with severe, chronic physical disorders such as immune dysfunction, hypertension, insulin resistance, abdominal obesity, atherosclerosis, osteoporosis, malnutrition, premenstrual syndrome, and hyperthyroidism.

It is also associated with behavioral and cognitive disorders such as anorexia nervosa, melancholic depression, long-term memory loss, panic disorder, obsessive-compulsive disorder, chronic active alcoholism, chronic excessive exercise, and vulnerability to addiction.[17][18][19]

On the other hand, chronically depressed stress system activity is also linked with physical and behavioral disorders. These include hypothyroidism, low-serotonin obesity, increased vulnerability to inflammatory and autoimmune diseases, atypical depression, chronic fatigue syndrome,

Cushing's syndrome, seasonal depression, post-traumatic stress disorder, and nicotine withdrawal.[20][21]

Since neither list is very appealing, you can see how important it is to find some simple "stress solutions" that can lower the risk of stress damage! Nutrition protection is an important key to stress protection, as you will see.

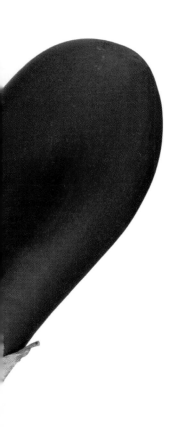

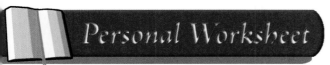

1. What types of stressors, if any, are dominant in my life? (see page 23)

Physical: —————————————————————————————

Emotional: —————————————————————————————

Chemical: —————————————————————————————

Environmental: —————————————————————————————

Symbolic: —————————————————————————————

Spiritual: —————————————————————————————

2. What symptoms, if any, am I experiencing that may be related to chronic stress? (see page 26)

———————————————————————————————————

———————————————————————————————————

———————————————————————————————————

3. Look up Psalm 32:8-9. What is the promise of God for every area of stress in my life? What is the condition?

———————————————————————————————————

———————————————————————————————————

———————————————————————————————————

4. Look up Psalm 33:11, Isaiah 45:19, and Isaiah 48:17. How trustworthy is the counsel of God, as revealed in the Bible? Is it good for today?

———————————————————————————————————

———————————————————————————————————

———————————————————————————————————

5. Look up Matthew 6:25-34. What do these verses say about priorities? What do these verses say about God's provision at all times?

———————————————————————————————————

———————————————————————————————————

———————————————————————————————————

(see answers on page 122)

Stress Effects on Nutrition

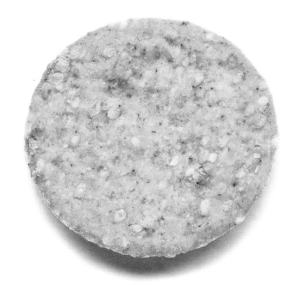

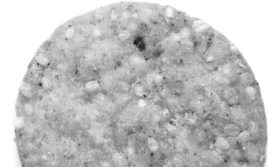

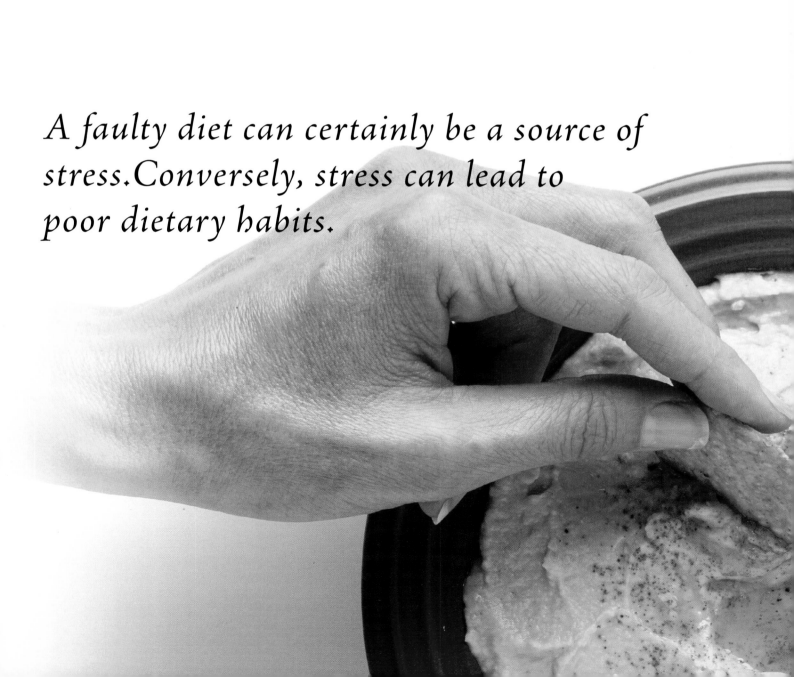

A faulty diet can certainly be a source of stress.Conversely, stress can lead to poor dietary habits.

Place in blender:

1 15-oz	Can garbanzo beans, drained or
	2 cups cooked garbanzos
¼ cup	Lemon juice
⅓ cup	Sesame tahini
2 tsp.	Garlic powder or
2	Cloves fresh garlic
1 tsp.	Salt
½ cup	Water

Serving Suggestions:

✦ This is a wholesome, versatile, quick, tasty recipe you'll want to eat often.

✦ Stuff it in a pita pocket with alfalfa sprouts, tomato, and green peppers for a delicious, nutritious sandwich.

✦ Place a generous scoop of it on your salad and squeeze fresh lemon on top.

✦ Put on baked potatoes with chives and olives.

✦ Use as a dip with chips or crackers.

✦ Stuff it in celery.

✦ For variety, add a stalk of celery, finely diced; and ¼ cup green onion, finely chopped.

> ## "We change, whether we like it or not."
> ~Ralph Waldo Emerson

You may be surprised to learn that you could be ignorantly bringing unnecessary stress into your life by your own lifestyle choices and habits. You may be even more surprised to learn that these same choices and habits make it more difficult to deal with the stressors that you can't escape!

In other words, not only does prolonged stress adversely affect nutritional status and needs, but your nutrition habits also affect how prone you are to stress, the intensity of your stress response, and your ability to cope with unavoidable stress![22] These facts illustrate how important it is to understand the relationship between nutrition and stress.

The better nourished you are, the better able you are to cope with stress. It is well known that changes take place in the levels of circulating hormones when stress occurs. The precise influence of a stress-altered metabolism on nutrient requirements is still being researched.[23] Some researchers have stated that almost any form of stress may influence nutritional balance.[24] This is because stress causes a general arousal that increases the body's metabolism, or the rate at which the body changes food supplies into energy.

> ## "Eating right is just as important as managing stress because vulnerability to stress increases with poor diet."
>
> Philip Rice, *Stress and Health.*
> Moorhead State University

Simply put, the body uses energy at a faster rate when stressed. According to Deborah Kipp, Ph.D., R.D., from the College of Health Sciences and Hospital in Kansas City, Kansas, "These changes, in turn, will influence the metabolism and, consequently, the requirements of nutrients."[25] Simply put, just as a speeding car needs more gas, a stressed body requires the right kind of nutrient "fuel."

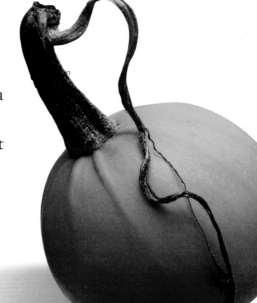

Prolonged stress increases the metabolic needs of the body because stress hormones tend to accelerate heart rate; increase muscle tension; elevate blood pressure, cholesterol, and triglyceride levels; and cause a cascade of other metabolic changes.[26] These changes increase metabolism and accelerate your body's use of carbohydrates, fats, and protein. As that usage changes, there can be a resulting increase in blood sugar, free fatty acids, and protein loss (negative nitrogen balance), respectively.[27] The increased metabolism can also cause an increase in the use and excretion of many nutrients such as vitamins A, C, D, E, K, and B complex, and minerals such as magnesium, calcium, phosphorus, chromium, selenium, zinc, and potassium.[28] But what happens if your body's "tank" is low on nutrition "fuel"?

While stress alters nutrient needs, if you are marginally deficient in a nutrient, stress can make that deficiency even worse! Bear in mind that poor nutrition or undernutrition is of itself a stress on the body. So when additional stress is imposed on the system, you will no longer have the same reserve capacity to adapt to the stress!

Vicious Stress Cycle

Unfortunately, it is often people who are the most easily stressed and in greatest need of a good diet, especially during times of extra stress, who make the worst food choices! This led researcher Paul Rosch to comment, "A faulty diet can certainly be a source of stress. Conversely, stress can lead to poor dietary habits."[29] Many people either stop eating almost entirely, or eat more frequently, shifting from well-planned, nourishing meals to junk food, fast food, alcohol, or stimulants such as caffeine or nicotine.

> **The effects of chronic stress may be exacerbated by a rich diet.**

Researchers who reviewed the factors that affect the stress response noted that: "The effects of chronic stress may be exacerbated by a rich diet."[30] Excess amounts of sugars and refined foods, for example, can diminish thiamine, niacin, B_{12}, magnesium, and calcium.[31] Low levels of these nutrients increase nervous-system reactivity, irritability, and nervousness.[32] But even more serious is the realization that poor eating habits in general lead to low concentrations of nutrients in the blood, which can impair brain function.[33]

Many depressed people crave sugary and/or fatty foods during stress. Yet increased sugar and fat consumption may be associated with the development or maintenance of depression.[34][35] Another vicious cycle!

On the other hand, a high-fiber diet rich in fresh fruits, vegetables, nuts, and whole grains provides greater appetite satisfaction over a longer period than processed, high-fat, and high-sugar snacks. But even more important, when you replace junk foods with fresh, high-fiber plant foods, you are more likely to consume greater amounts of vitamins A, B_6, and C, and the B vitamins niacin, thiamin, riboflavin, and folate. You will also have a higher intake of magnesium, iron, selenium, zinc, phosphorus, and calcium.[36] These nutrients are all vital to a healthy metabolism and provide significant stress protection. One study of food and mood concluded that, "Overall, the results suggest that a dietary change can remediate the emotional stress exhibited by some individuals."[37]

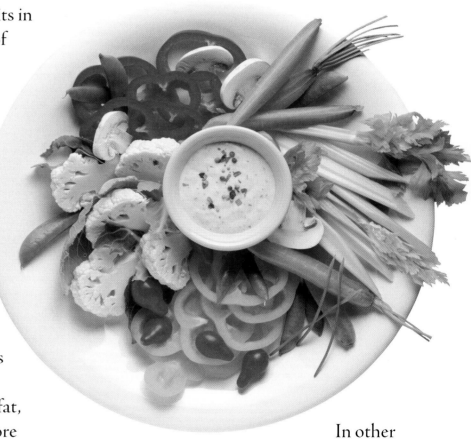

In other words, improving your quality of food choices can help you to reduce stress effects!

Vitamins &

VITAMINS

A

vegetables—dark green & yellow
fruits—dark green & yellow

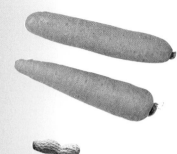

B$_1$

whole grains—wheat germ, oatmeal
nuts—cashews, peanuts, pecans, walnuts
vegetables—most

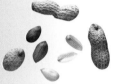

B$_2$

whole grains—wheat bran,
enriched cornmeal, soyflour
nutritional yeast (Red Star T-6635)
nuts
vegetables—green leafy

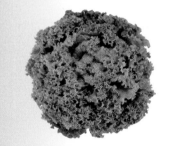

B$_5$

legumes—dried beans and peas, peanuts
whole grains—wheat germ
yeast
vegetables—dark green

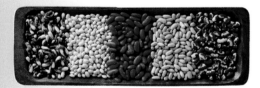

B$_6$

nutritional yeast (Red Star T-6635)
nuts, seeds—sunflower, sesame
whole grains
vegetables—many, especially leafy vegetables
blackstrap molasses

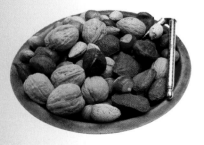

&*Minerals*

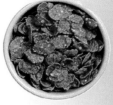

B$_{12}$

strict vegetarians require a
fortified source, such as
supplements, or fortified foods like
ready-to-eat cereal
nutritional yeast (Red Star T-6635)

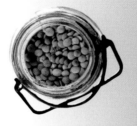

Niacin

whole grain products
fortified cereals
nuts—peanuts
vegetables—green, potatoes
legumes

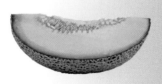

Folic acid

vegetables—dark green leafy
whole grains—breakfast cereals, yeast
legumes—lentils
nuts
fruits—citrus

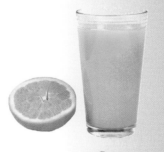

C

fruit—citrus, berries, cantaloupe
vegetables—green peppers, broccoli,
cauliflower, green leafy vegetables,
cabbage, potatoes

D

sunshine on a regular basis
fortified foods—soy and other
milks, fortified cereals, fortified
orange juice

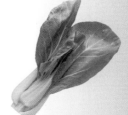

E

nuts
whole grain—cereals, wheat germ
vegetables—green leafy
vegetable oils – soybean, safflower, sunflower

K

cereals - some
vegetables – green leafy (spinach,
lettuce, kale, cabbage), cauliflower, small
amounts in other vegetables
soybean oil
synthesized by bacteria in the intestine

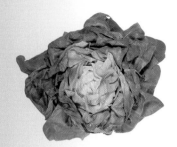

MINERALS:

Calcium

green leafy vegetables (collard greens, chard,
beet tops, Bok Choy,
spinach and broccoli)
seeds, almonds
beans - soybeans, calcium-prepared tofu
lime-prepared corn tortillas, fortified vegan milks
fortified cereals
figs

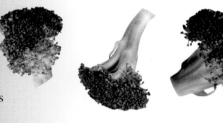

Chromium

whole grain – cereals, breads,
nutritional yeast (Red Star T-6635)
vegetables – whole potatoes,
beets, vegetables grown in
chromium rich soil
grape juice
beans
stainless steel cookware used with acid foods

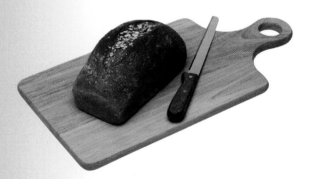

Iron

whole grains—oatmeal, brown rice,
wheat germ, fortified flour, fortified cereal
blackstrap molasses
dark leafy green vegetables
nuts, seeds (sunflower seeds)
soybeans, legumes
Fruits—dried fruits (raisins, figs, prunes, dates,
dried apricots), blackberries, cherries,
watermelon
(vitamin C increases uptake, as does
yeasted bread versus unyeasted—the
polyphenols in tea and coffee inhibit iron
absorption)

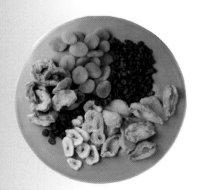

Magnesium

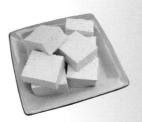

green vegetables
magnesium-based tofu
whole grains—bran, wheat germ, amaranth
seeds, nuts
beans, soybeans

Potassium

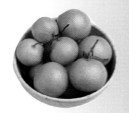

fruits—bananas, cantaloupe,
grapefruit, watermelon, dried fruit, avocado,
dried peas and beans,
vegetables - baked potato, winter squash,
brussels sprouts, mustard greens

Selenium

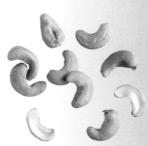

whole grains
nuts—Brazil nuts, cashews

Zinc

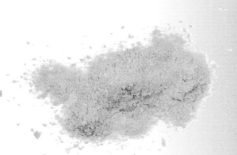

whole grains, bran, nutritional yeast
legumes—beans, soybeans
nuts & seeds—sunflower seeds, nuts
vegetables—spinach, peas
(vitamin C increases uptake, as does yeasted
bread). Also the polyphenols
in tea and coffee inhibit
absorption. Excessive copper, calcium,
and iron displace zinc and limit uptake

Vitamins and Minerals that are Altered as a Result of Stress

Decreased		Increased
Vitamins	**Minerals**	**Minerals**
A	Calcium	Sodium
C	Chromium	Chloride
D	Iron	Copper
E	Magnesium	
K	Phosphorus	
B_1	Potassium	
B_2	Zinc	
B_5		
B_6		
B_{12}		
Niacin		
Folic Acid		

Source: Asterita, Mary F. Ph.D. "Physical Exercise, Nutrition and Stress" Table 10.3, p. 145

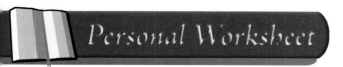

1. Am I involved in "emotional eating," i.e, eating out of anger, frustration, stress, depression, etc., but not hunger? What types of foods and drinks do I turn to when I am feeling stressed?

    _____

    _____

    _____

2. Look up Psalm 142:1-5. What is a better solution than food when feeling overwhelmed?

    _____

    _____

    _____

3. Look up Proverbs 26:27. Why does God want me to reason from cause to effect in my daily choices?

    _____

    _____

    _____

4. Look up Luke 21:34. How is uncontrolled behavior especially risky at the end of time? ("surfeiting" means gluttony)

    _____

    _____

    _____

5. Look up Proverbs 25:16 and 30:8-9. What are the two greatest dangers of uncontrolled appetite, even of good foods?

    _____

    _____

    _____

(see answers on page 122)

Nutrition Effects on Stress

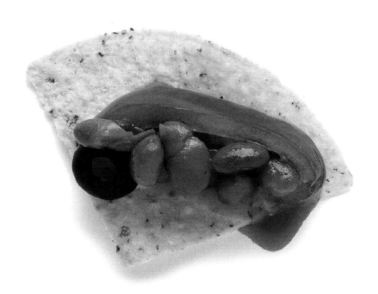

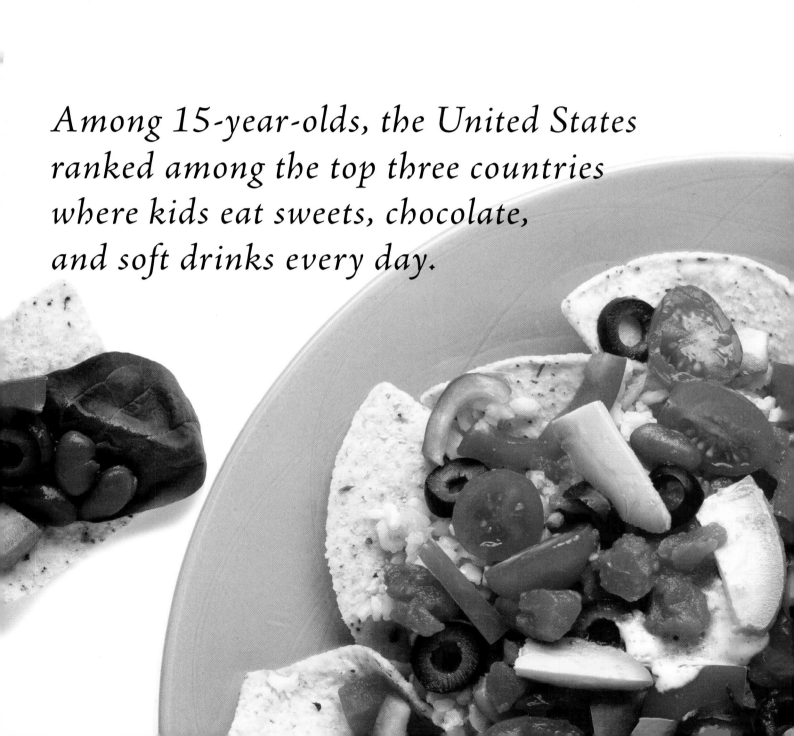

Among 15-year-olds, the United States ranked among the top three countries where kids eat sweets, chocolate, and soft drinks every day.

Haystacks are a version of a taco salad where you "build your own plate."

Easy Oven Brown Rice
2 cups water
1 cup brown rice
Place in baking dish. Cover. Bake at 350° for 1 to 1½ hours.

Easy Beans
Saute onion. Add canned beans—pinto, black, red, or chili. Add your choice of seasonings: onion powder, garlic powder, paprika.

Build your haystack.

Place on a plate:
Brown rice and/or baked chips

Add:
Your choice of beans or chili

Then add your choice of:
Shredded lettuce
Chopped tomatoes
Chopped green onions
Sliced olives
Diced avocado
Chopped bell peppers

Top with:
Creamy Cheese Sauce (see recipe on p. 22)
Salsa
And/or tofu sour cream

Serving Suggestions

✦ This is great for a quick meal or to serve when you have a large group of people.

"The heaviest rains fall on the leaky house."
~Japanese saying

Lifestyle choices affect both mind and body. As early as 300 B.C. the Greek surgeon and anatomist Herophilus wrote: "When health is absent, wisdom cannot reveal itself, art cannot become manifest, strength cannot be exerted, wealth is useless, and reason is powerless."

Isn't it odd that many people ruin their health the first half of their life trying to make more money, and then spend the second half of their life spending money trying to get their health back!

For many people, mealtime is fast, frenzied, and often "thawed-out" instead of "thought-out."

For many Americans today, the basic four food groups are "nuked," canned, boxed, and "fast." In short, it is unbalanced, unhealthful, unsatisfying, and unnatural! Can good mental or physical health be the result of such poor, haphazard choices?

"Increased daily ingestion of caffeine is associated with higher levels of anxiety symptoms in both healthy and psychiatric patients."
Arc Gen Psychiatry 1985; 42: 233-243

"Rushing" Roulette?

Are you chowing down on fat- and sugar-laden foods such as pizzas and fries, pastries and pies, chips, chops, and lollipops, and turning away from hundreds of power-packed, tasty, easy-to-fix fresh fruits, nuts, vegetables, whole grains, and legumes? America is gulping down this fiberless fare with a national daily ration of 33 million gallons of coffee per day. That is the equivalent of 30 seconds full flow of water over Niagara Falls! But all that coffee isn't quenching our thirst. Americans drink an average of 547 cans of soda pop per person per year (643 in the South), at a total cost of 47.3 billion dollars! And it's not just the cans that are getting bigger—so are our problems! Is it possible that our "revved-up" diet is contributing to a "stressed-out" America?

By conservative estimates, up to 30 percent of adult Americans have a daily caffeine intake of more than 500 mg.[38] Caffeine is a drug that temporarily increases the sensation of alertness, but research has shown that over time caffeine may increase stress-sensitivity, anxiety, and depression. It can also encourage the loss of nutrients such as calcium, magnesium, and B vitamins.[39][40] But the most subtle and devastating long-term effect of caffeine may be its slow erosion of vital nerve centers in the brain that balance stress hormone levels. This can eventually affect memory and risk of depression. How? Caffeine causes an elevation of a stress hormone called cortisol. Cortisol can accumulate in a brain memory center called the hippocampus.[41] The hippocampus is essential for short-term memory and is also a key player in regulation of your body's stress system.

When cortisol levels remain too high for too long from exposure to chronic stress or chemical stimulation such as caffeine, cell death can occur in the hip-pocampus, as well as other vital areas of the brain.[42] The result can include memory impairment, chronic depression, and chronic "dysregulation" of the stress system.

Coffee, tea, and soft drink consumption tend to cause vitamin and mineral loss and dehydration. According to the American Dietetic Association, dehydration of as little as two percent loss of body weight can reduce your mental and physical abilities. Plentiful water intake (about eight glasses a day for a typical adult) reduces sluggishness by enhancing circulation and enabling your blood to carry life and energy-giving nutrients to the body's cells!

Sweet Stressors

Carbohydrates are needed to increase the brain's uptake of tryptophan. Tryptophan is essential for the production of serotonin, a hormone that helps regulate mood, appetite, pain tolerance, food cravings, and sleep. It has been suggested that many "sugar-holics" are actually self-medicating due to the mood-elevating effects of increased serotonin. If so, there's a lot of medicating going on, from babyhood up! Some experts estimate that the average adult intake of refined

Filled Out or Filled Up?

Equal Calories

High-Fat, Low-Fiber	Low-Fat, High-Fiber

High-Fat, Low-Fiber

- 1 8-oz. chocolate bar
- 1 5-oz. chocolate bar
- 1 cheeseburger
- 1 danish
- 1 slice chocolate cake
- 1 milkshake
- 1 peanut butter parfait
- 5-oz. steak
- 12 marshmallows
- 1/2 cup peanuts
- 6 small chocolate chip cookies

Fills You OUT:

Low-Fat, High-Fiber

- 25 carrots
- 3 pounds apples
- 21 cups popcorn
- apple, banana, orange & ½ cantaloupe
- 7 slices whole wheat bread
- 5 bananas
- 7 bananas
- 5 baked potatoes
- 60 stalks of celery
- 600 cucumber slices
- 20 green peppers, 3 ears of corn

Fills You UP!

sweeteners (sucrose and fructose) is about 120 lbs. per person per year. In analyzing the diets of 15,000 Americans aged two and older, it was found that table sugar and sweeteners in processed foods account for nearly one-fifth, or 20 percent, of American's carbohydrate intake.[43]

In two- to five-year-olds, sugars, candy, and sweetened fruit drinks were major sources of carbohydrates, followed by soft drinks. In the six to 11 age group, soft drinks, sweetened cereals, cakes, cookies, and sweetened fruit drinks were

> *In two- to five-year olds, sugars, candy, and sweetened fruit drinks were major sources of carbohydrates, followed by soft drinks.*

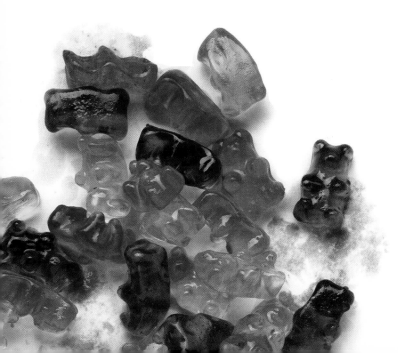

the favorites. In teens, almost four-tenths, or 40 percent, of sugar calories came from soft drinks![44] Among 15-year-olds, the United States ranked among the top three countries where kids eat sweets, chocolate, and soft drinks every day![45]

The problem is, there is a down-side to the quick lift associated with low-fiber, refined sweets. While it is true that simple carbohydrates elevate serotonin levels, they elevate them only for a short time.[46] Repeated ingestion of quick "pick-me-up" snacks that are low in real nutrition not only play havoc with hormones but also with blood sugar, insulin, and blood nutrient levels. They are a real "downer" when it comes to stress protection.

Your body needs carbohydrates for energy. But the best form of energy is the slow-releasing carbs found in whole grains such as whole wheat bread, oats, whole grain pasta, beans, unrefined potatoes, unrefined cereals, and brown rice. These provide sustained energy and hundreds of phytochemicals, vitamins, and minerals vital to physical and mental health. In fact, complex carbohydrates or starch foods with natural fiber and nutrient constituents result in longer, more sustained levels of brain serotonin.[47] It is no surprise, then, that those who consume breakfast cereal regularly report better mental and physical health than those who consume it infrequently.[48]

Is There a Tiger in Your Tank?

As the proportion of meals eaten away from home has nearly doubled in the last twenty years,[49] meat and animal protein foods are taking a lion's share of daily energy intake. Is the lion's alternately groggy then irritable disposition the price tag for such "copycat" eating?

Very high protein diets are popular today, but while the benefits are doubtful at best, they may increase stress sensitivity. According to one study, individuals with high-stress proneness had more energy and lower stress proneness after a meal high in carbohydrates and low in protein than after a meal high in protein and low in carbohydrates.[50] High-protein, low-carbohydrate diets are associated with worse performance on mental flexibility tasks and higher levels of irritability, anxiety, and depression.[51] [52]

One reason may be that very high protein diets tend to be high in the amino acid tyrosine. Tyrosine is necessary for the important brain hormones dopamine and norepinephrine, which help elevate mood and energy. But if tyrosine levels are very high at every meal, then serotonin

Nuts, beans, legumes, soy, seeds, and whole grains are excellent sources of plant-based protein... and are also rich sources of minerals, vitamins, and phytochemicals.

levels drop, and low serotonin is associated with depression, eating disorders, and insomnia, among other problems. We need protein in the diet, but excessive amounts just may set your nerves on edge. The key word here is balance.

It is a popular notion that if you want to be alert, load up on protein, and if you want to be calm, eat plenty of "carbs." While it is true that these foods can have a short-term effect on mental alertness and perhaps even mood, meals that are consistently balanced in their protein, carbohydrates, and fat are the best overall plan for long-term stress protection and consistent mental strength.

The long-term effects associated with diets high in meat and dairy

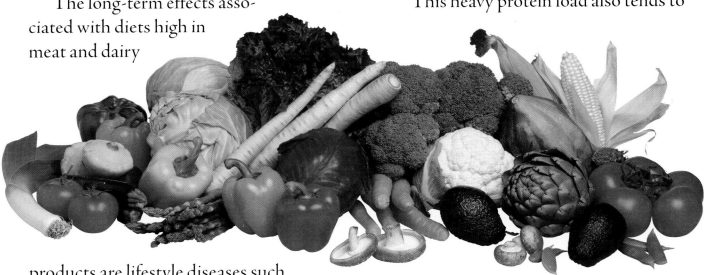

products are lifestyle diseases such as heart disease, elevated cholesterol, high blood pressure, and Type II diabetes. It is interesting that these diseases are also associated with cognitive impairment and an increased risk for dementia.[53] There are serious health consequences to dietary habits that "stress" the metabolism over long periods of time.

The typical American diet, loaded with meats, cheeses, eggs, and other animal protein, is no stress-reliever and can quickly rack up a daily protein load of 120 grams or more! Less than half that much is all that is needed for most adults (45 grams for women, and 55 grams for men). A day's menu that includes just one chicken breast, an eight-ounce burger, two ounces of cheese, and one cup of yogurt adds up to 120 grams of protein! These inordinately high protein diets tend to deprive the brain of carbohydrates and antioxidants, which are needed for proper function and maintenance.

This heavy protein load also tends to overwork the kidneys, leach calcium from the bones, and create metabolic stress that promotes inflammatory diseases and cardiovascular disease. Nuts, beans, legumes, soy, seeds, and whole grains are excellent sources of plant-based protein, which are metabolically more "user friendly" and are also rich sources of minerals, vitamins, and phytochemicals.

A plant-based vegetarian diet, containing adequate calories and a good variety of protein foods such as grains, beans, nuts, tofu, and legumes in the menu for the week, will provide all the protein necessary for a healthful, balanced diet, without tipping the protein scale on the wrong side. Add to this delicious variety your choice of hearty, fiber-filled complex carbohydrates such as potatoes, yams, squash, and plenty of fresh fruits and leafy green vegetables. Include a little olive oil, some avocado, olives, or nuts for healthful fats, and you have a balanced and beautiful mix of foods that will calm your nerves while strengthening your mental faculties!

Lowering Stress...

"Who hath despised the day of small things?"

Zechariah 4:10

One Bite at a Time!

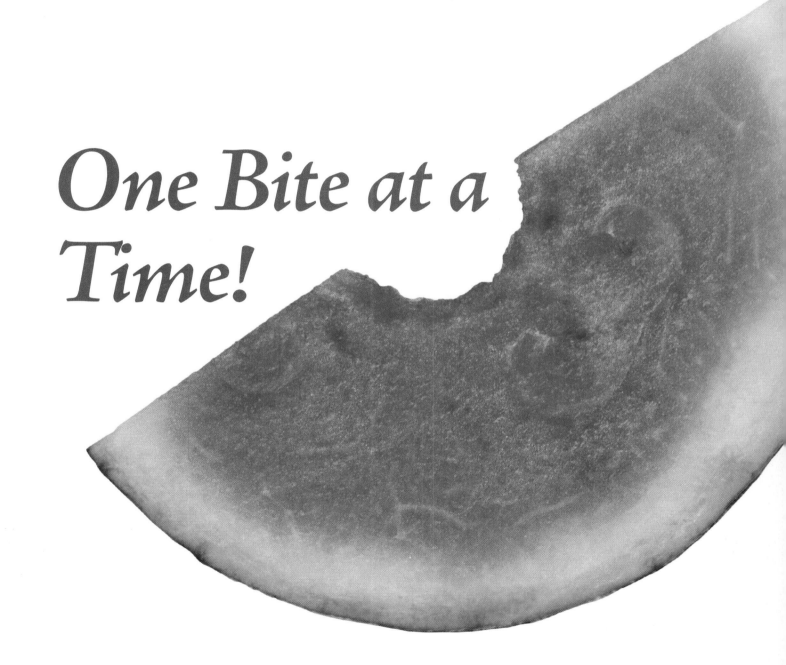

Breakfast

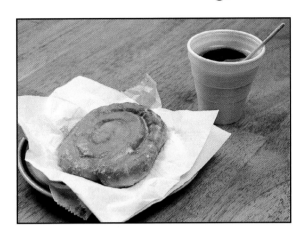

Instead of:

Coffee

Danish

What Have You

Caffeine—facts and effects:
- ✦ dehydration, irritability;
- ✦ increase in stress hormones, artificial stimulation;
- ✦ potential loss of calcium, magnesium, B-vitamins;
- ✦ elevates insulin and triglycerides which may complicate heart health and diabetes;
- ✦ increased stomach acidity.

Danish—facts and effects:
- ✦ approximately 200 calories of refined sugar and unhealthy fats;
- ✦ limited vitamins and minerals;
- ✦ high sugar and saturated and trans fat content may cause calcium, magnesium and B-vitamin loss;
- ✦ the type of fats in the danish may intensify stress sensitivity;
- ✦ low fiber content contributes to "rush" of energy followed by low energy mood;
- ✦ low fiber content doesn't satisfy, so hunger occurs soon after eating.

Better Breakfast

Try:

Two cups water upon arising
  (*30 minutes later*)

Two fresh fruits

Whole wheat toast with nut butter
  and applesauce

Fortified soy or other milk

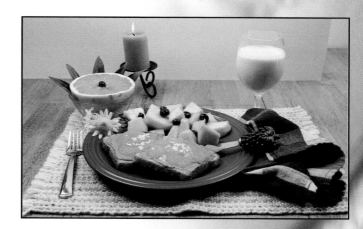

Accomplished?

Benefits of water:
- ✦ hydrates your body, increases nutrient and oxygen flow to the brain;
- ✦ enhances alertness naturally—wakes you up and gets you going;
- ✦ aids in digestion, absorption and utilization of nutrients.

Benefits of fresh fruit:
- ✦ satisfies your sweet tooth, with low calorie, healthy energy source;
- ✦ provides rich matrix of fiber, vitamins, minerals, phytochemicals and water to protect against stress;
- ✦ aids digestion, satisfies hunger;
- ✦ as part of a total meal, protects against swings in blood sugar levels.

Benefits of whole wheat toast, almond butter, applesauce, fortified soy milk:
- ✦ supply a balance of protein, carbohydrate and fat for energy and cellular building blocks;
- ✦ provide a better quality of fat that benefits the brain and nervous system;
- ✦ add vital nutrients such as selenium, magnesium, calcium, chromium, thiamin, and small amounts of other B-vitamins and vitamin D;
- ✦ the fiber content will provide satiety and reduce the urge to snack;
- ✦ the complex carbohydrates will increase mood elevating, calming hormones in the brain;
- ✦ sources of disease-fighting, brain-enhancing antioxidants.

Lunch

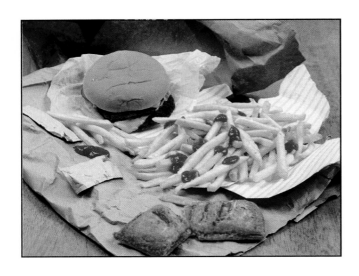

Instead of:

Burger
Fries
Apple pie

What Have You

Burger and fries—facts and effects:
- ✦ high in pro-inflammatory, pro-stress fats;
- ✦ low in fiber;
- ✦ low in nutrients, low in plant antioxidants;
- ✦ can cause after-lunch dip in energy, increased sleepiness;
- ✦ can impair blood flow and reduce oxygen to brain;
- ✦ can elevate insulin levels and blood fats.

Apple pie—facts and effects:
- ✦ similar effects as the burger and fries;
- ✦ refined sugar may increase tension and fatigue;
- ✦ calorie overload can elevate triglycerides.

Luscious Lunch

Try:

Whole wheat bread with
   hummus, tomato slices, leaf
   lettuce, bell pepper slices

And:

Carrot and celery sticks, and a few
nuts with dates or figs for dessert

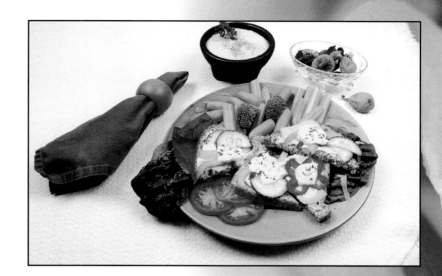

Accomplished?

Benefits of vegetables, and hummus* on whole wheat bread:
+ rich source of fiber, digestive enzymes, antioxidants;
+ stress-lowering greens provide phytochemicals, vitamins, and minerals;
+ satisfy hunger and provide calming carotenoids;
+ aid digestion, promote regularity and gut health.

Benefits of nuts and dates:
+ healthy and delicious dessert which satisfies desire for sweets and fats;
+ healthy fat promotes health of nervous system and brain;
+ fiber slows release of carbohydrates into system;
+ source of anti-stress minerals such as selenium, magnesium, and calcium.

* Hummus is a spread made from garbanzo beans that can be purchased at
most stores in the refrigerated produce section, or see the easy recipe in
   this book *(page 34)*.

Supper

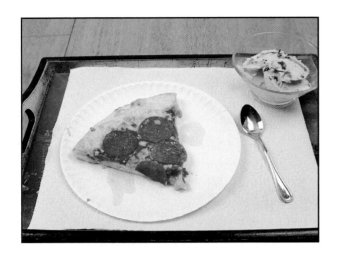

Instead of:

Pizza
Ice cream

What Have You

Pizza and ice cream—facts and effects:

+ rich, unhealthy fat- and refined sugar-dense meal is pro-stress;
+ hard to digest, especially at night—impairs restful sleep;
+ high saturated and trans fat with high sugar can impair concentration;
+ low in fiber, nutrients, and antioxidants;
+ excess fat and sugar can cause loss of stored nutrients;
+ high-calorie load at night contributes to obesity.

Sumptuous Supper

Try:

Vegetable soup with whole grain crackers

And:

Air-popped pop corn seasoned with olive oil, onion powder, and salt

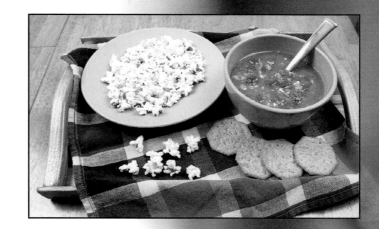

Accomplished?

Benefits of vegetable soup, crackers, and air-popped popcorn:

- ✦ lower calorie, nutrient-rich foods better for evening meal;
- ✦ higher fiber content promotes regularity, protects against obesity;
- ✦ rich source of nutrients, antioxidants, and other stress-protective compounds;
- ✦ satisfying but easier to digest than heavy, animal-based meal;
- ✦ fat used on popcorn is healthier for the brain and heart.

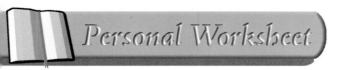

1. Which foods and drinks am I consuming on a regular basis that may be contributing to stress, depression, fatigue, and irritability in my life?

_____

_____

_____

2. Which foods can I start adding to my diet to replace unhealthy choices that will help lower stress levels, and improve my mood and energy levels?

_____

_____

_____

3. List the types of foods that need to be in my diet every day.

_____

_____

_____

4. Look up Genesis 1:29 and Genesis 2:9, 16. What was God's original diet for men and women at creation? How much were Adam and Eve to eat?

_____

_____

_____

5. Look up Daniel 1:12. When the prophet Daniel was in captivity in Babylon, under extreme pressure, what diet did he request? ("Pulse" means vegetables.)

_____

_____

_____

(see answers on page 123)

Fretting About Fat?

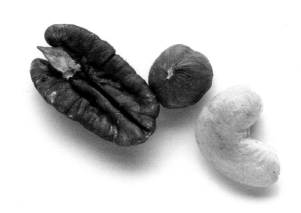
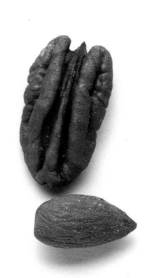
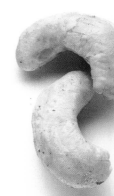

*We need fat in the diet,
especially the type of fat
found in nuts, olives,
avocados, olive
oil, and seeds.*

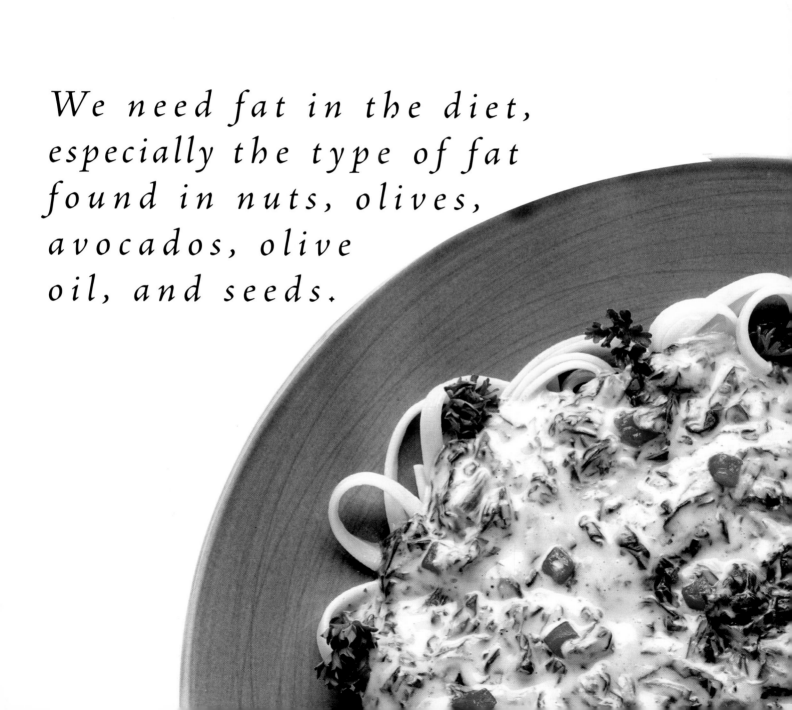

8-oz	Fettuccini noodles
4	Garlic cloves. crushed
1 tsp.	Salt
1 tsp.	Basil
1 tsp.	Onion powder
1 box	Tofu, silken, 12.5oz
2 cups	Soy or rice milk (plain)
2 T	Flour
2 cups	Spinach, chopped/frozen, thawed, and well-drained
⅓ cup	Parsley, fresh

Cook noodles in salted water until tender. Drain. In a separate pan, saute spinach and garlic in ¼ cup water for about 2 minutes. Add salt, basil, onion powder, and parsley. Blend tofu, milk and flour in a blender. Pour into spinach mixture. Cook 2 more minutes. Toss with noodles. Add a little olive oil for flavor. Garnish with pimientos, if desired.

✦ **Serves 8.**

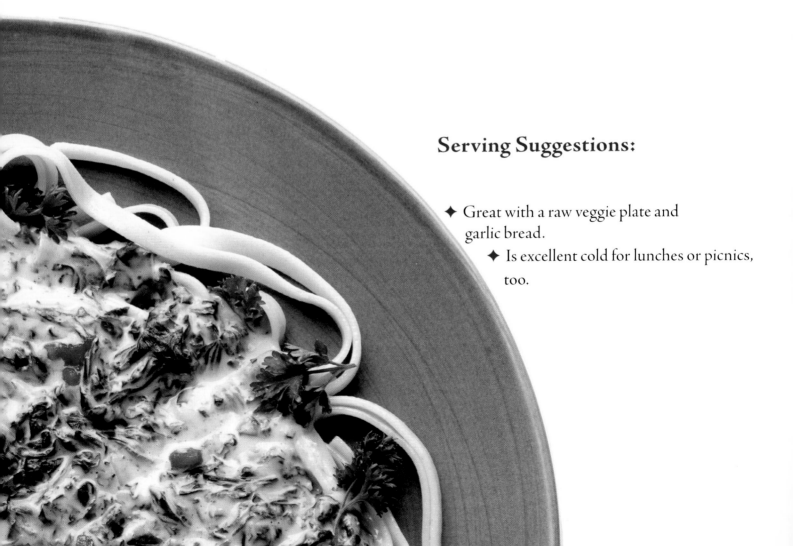

Serving Suggestions:

✦ Great with a raw veggie plate and garlic bread.

✦ Is excellent cold for lunches or picnics, too.

We need fat in the diet, especially the type of fat found in nuts, olives, avocados, olive oil, and seeds.

A diet too high in protein is not the only potential stress intensifier. The typical American diet is high in saturated animal fat (animal products, eggs) and omega 6 fats (vegetable oils such as corn, safflower, and peanut), hydrogenated and partially hydrogenated fats (margarine, vegetable shortening, french fries, commercially baked products such as corn and potato chips, pastries, and crackers). A diet rich in these foods is also associated with intensification of the stress response. Consider this: "Diets relatively rich in long-chain fatty acids…as well as diets very rich in relatively saturated long-chain fatty acids may cause magnification of stress reactions."[54] Simply put, some types of fat, when taken in large amounts, tend to stress you out!

Indeed, one study on dietary fat intake concluded: "Dietary fat intake acts as a background form of chronic stress," causing the elevation of several stress hormones.[55] Another study demonstrated that "stress responsivity is briefly enhanced during initial access to the high-fat regimens. Continued

high-fat feeding results in an impaired ability to restore basal [normal] corticosterone [stress hormones] following

"Dietary fat acts as a background form of chronic stress."

Am J Physiol, 1997;273 (6 Pt. 1):E1168-77.

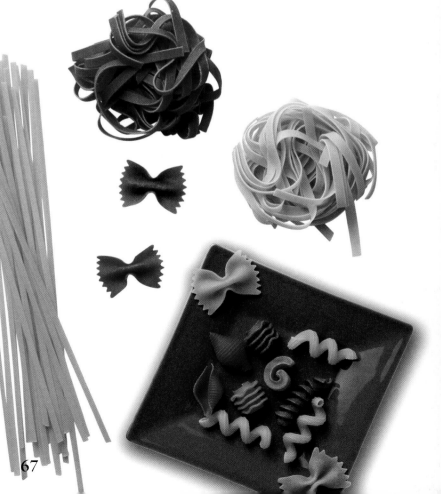

67

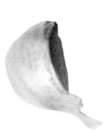

stress."[56] Translated into easy English: high-fat diets make you stressed-out and keep you stressed-out longer!

Friendly Fats

So should we be distressed about all fats? No! We need fat in the diet, especially the type of fat found in nuts, olives, avocados, olive oil, and seeds (the omega-3 and monounsaturated type fats, or MUFAs). Even though most fat sources contain combinations of several types of fats including saturated and omega-6 fats, these foods contain higher proportions of the types of fats that are good for the brain and nervous system. Remember, all fat sources are concentrated sources of calories, so weight, activity level, and age must be taken into consideration when planning meals. Recommendations for consumption of these healthier fats vary from 25 percent to 40 percent. But remember, overloading the system with too many calories even from

healthy fats and carbohydrates can lead to obesity and other problems.

Omega-3 fats are thought to have an antidepressive and calming effect on the nervous system, and MUFAs are important, especially for the aging brain. If you're like most Americans, you need more of these types of fats and less of the unhealthful fats found in processed foods.[57] But a diet rich in animal fat and

A diet rich in animal fat and trans fatty acids can stimulate the production of stress hormones.

polyunsaturated fats (such as cooking oils, margarine, etc.), are can stimulate the production of stress hormones.[58]

The animal source of fat that is an exception to the above is fish, which is a source of omega-3 fats plus preformed fatty acids such as EPA and DHA. But your body makes EPA and DHA from the plant sources of omega-3 that you eat. Plant sources of omega-3 fatty acids may be preferable for several reasons. First, fish oil capsules may be concentrated sources of vitamin A and D, which can be toxic in large doses.

Second, pesticides and contaminants such as polychlorinated biphenyls (PCBs) and dioxin are concentrated in the fatty tissue of fish and the fatty tissues of those who consume them. Women who live in Scandinavian countries eat diets high in fish and high-fat dairy products. The high level of PCB's and dioxins in their diets have given rise to subtle abnormalities in nursing newborns such as disturbed cognitive development and delayed motor development.[59] Another source of PCB and dioxin exposure besides fish products and high-fat dairy products is beef.[60] New research indicates that adult exposure to these compounds is associated with impairment in learning and memory.[61]

Third, mercury contamination is a serious issue. A recent analysis of 53,000 records of mercury test results in fish from numerous federal, state, and other government sources led Jane Houlihan, principal author of a report issued by the U.S. Public Interest Research Group, to comment, "The widespread contamination of fish with mercury has given its reputation as 'brain food' a new and disturbing connotation because fetal exposure to mercury can lead to learning deficiencies and may delay mental development in children."[62] Her recommendation: limit most types of fish intake to once a month for pregnant women.

Fourth, commercially fed fish such as salmon and trout are often very low in omega-3 fatty acid and higher in saturated and omega-6 fats. Interestingly, these fish tend to develop cardiovascular disease![63]

Stress Savers

In addition to diet, there are a few other simple lifestyle stress-savers that can help sweeten up your mood, roll away stress, and energize your life.

Water

Two of the first signs of mild dehydration are irritability and fatigue. Drink plenty of fresh water between meals, instead of dehydrating sodas and caffeinated drinks. Eight glasses a day will help your mental engine "purr" instead of "ping!"

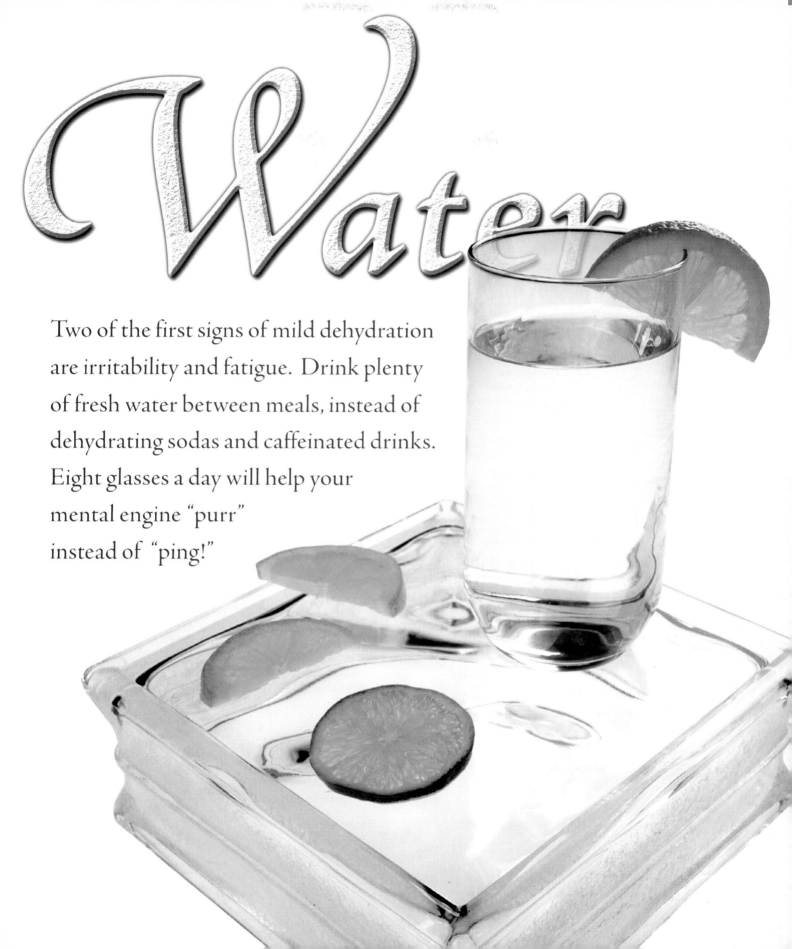

Exercise

Just a 10-minute brisk walk can boost your mood for up to one hour, but a sugary or fatty snack will ultimately increase feelings of tension and fatigue. Just 30 minutes of exercise a day can have a major anti-stress impact on your life!

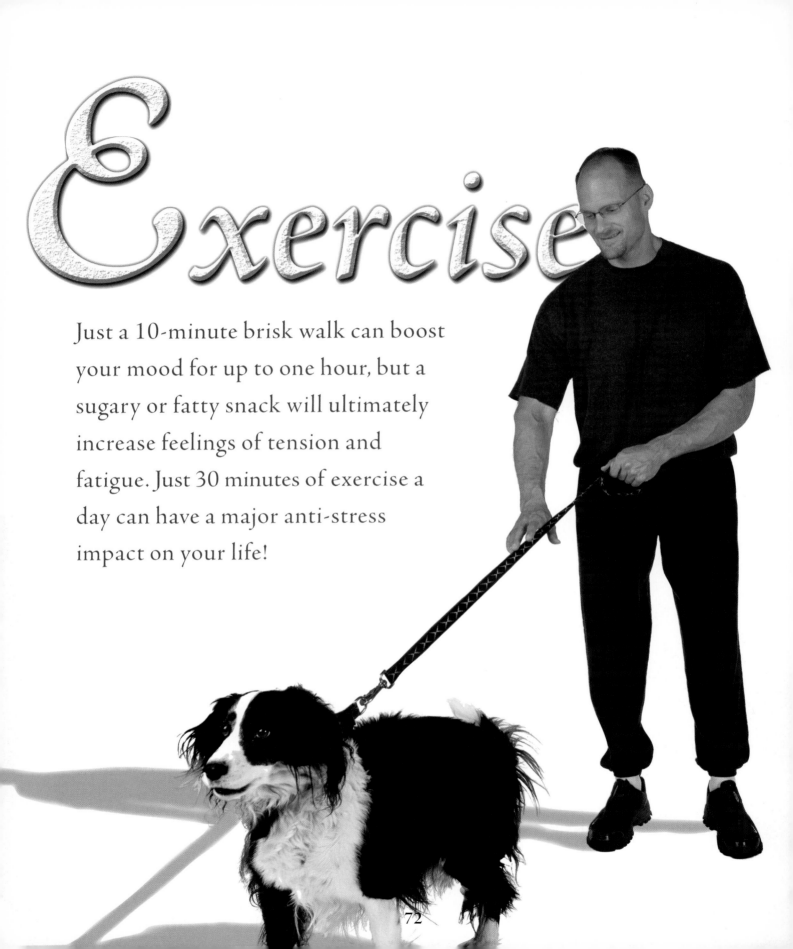

Sleep

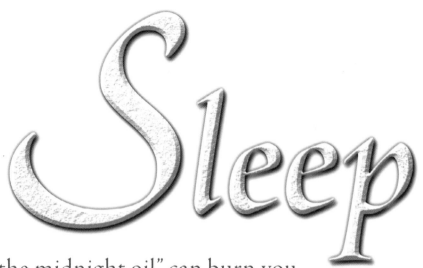

"Burning the midnight oil" can burn you out, especially your stress system. Getting to bed at least 2 or 3 hours before midnight improves mood and performance the next day. It also improves blood sugar control and lowers stress hormone production.

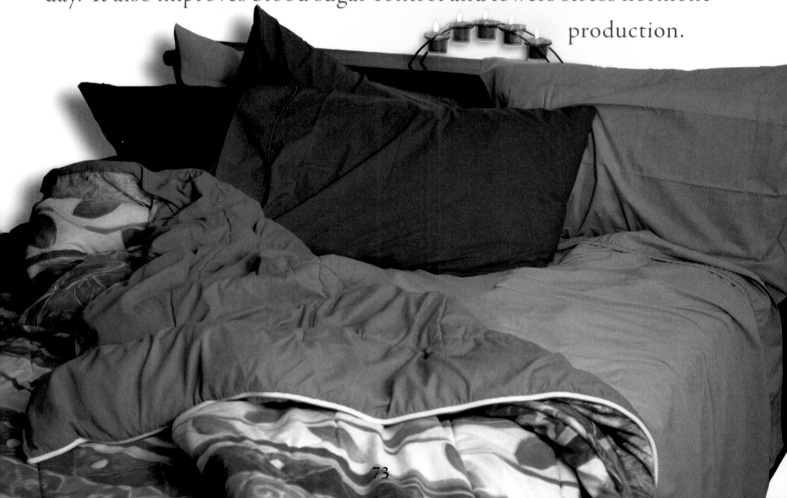

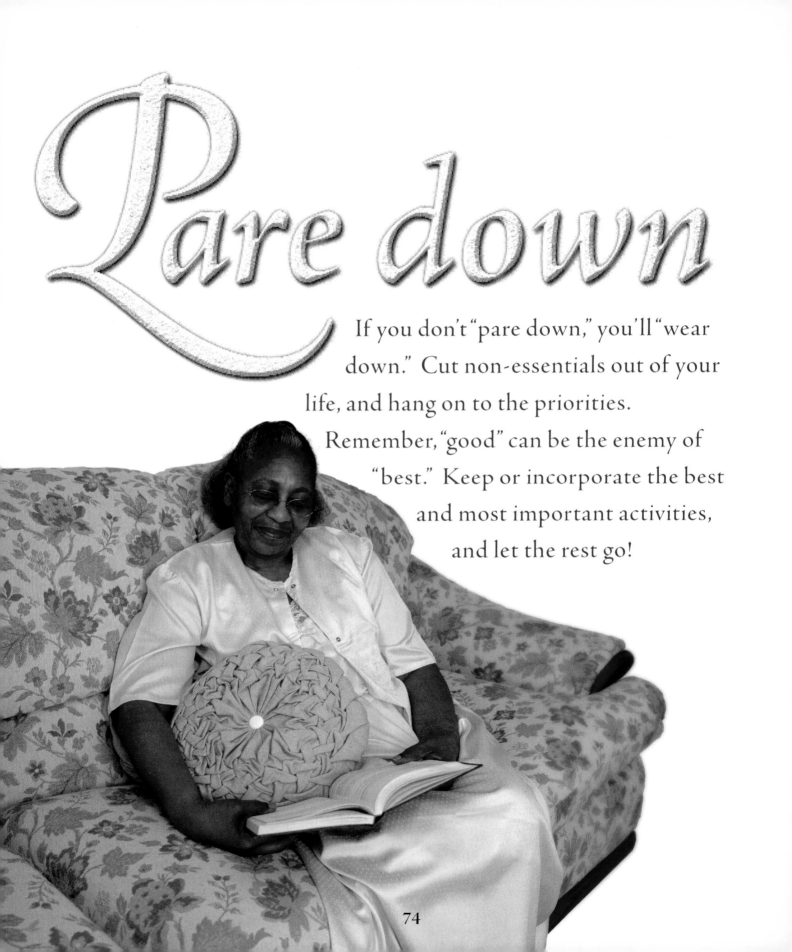

Pare down

If you don't "pare down," you'll "wear down." Cut non-essentials out of your life, and hang on to the priorities. Remember, "good" can be the enemy of "best." Keep or incorporate the best and most important activities, and let the rest go!

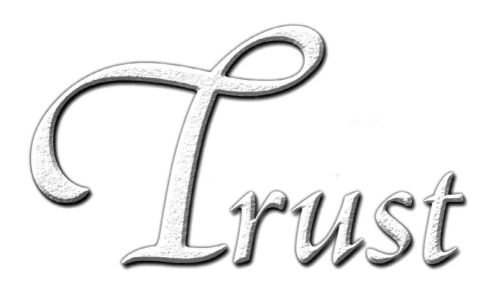

Trust

Spiritual well-being is at the center of a healthy lifestyle. The Bible tells us, "Be anxious for nothing, but in everything by prayer ... let your requests be made known to God. And the peace of God, which passes all understanding, shall keep your hearts and minds through Christ Jesus." Philippians 4:6-7. A Friend to help in every need— now that's stress relief!

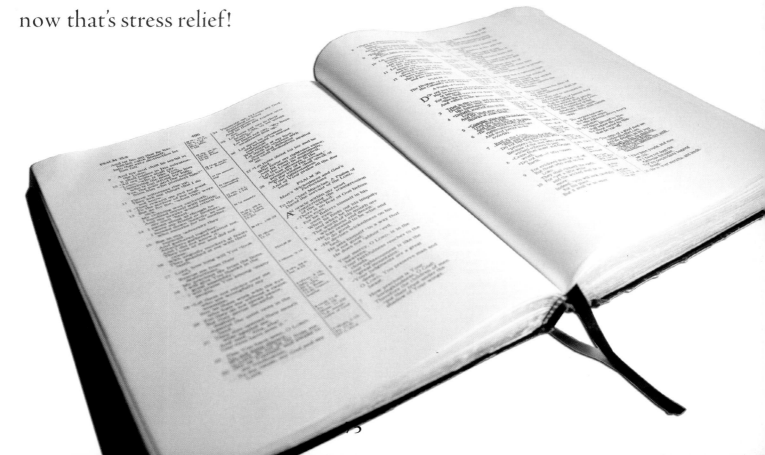

Personal Worksheet

1. What are the major sources of fat in my diet?

_____

_____

_____

2. What "healthy fats" are accessible to me?

_____

_____

_____

3. Look up Isaiah 24:4-6. What is foretold regarding the condition of the earth (including the animal kingdom) at the end of earth's history? Why?

_____

_____

_____

4. Look up Proverbs 23:20-21. What is the counsel regarding the excessive use of flesh? What is the result?

_____

_____

_____

5. How can I include healthy fats into my meals?

Breakfast: _____

Lunch: _____

Supper: _____

(see answers on page 123)

Plants or Pills?

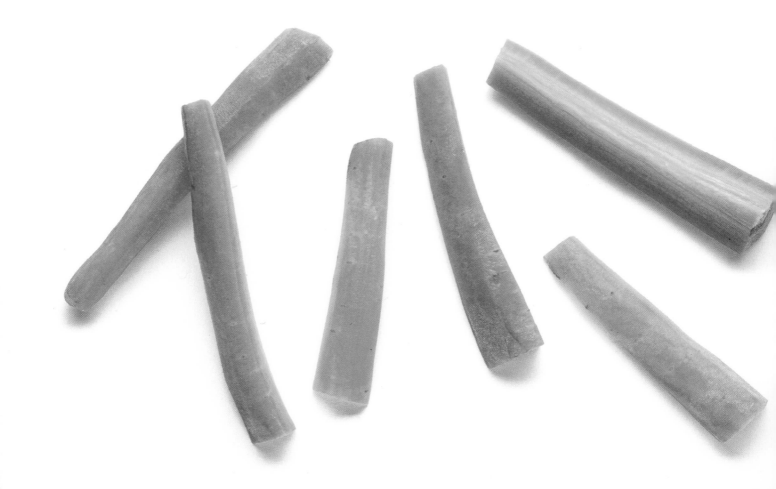

Consumers spend almost four billion dollars annually on more than 40,000 different vitamin and mineral products.

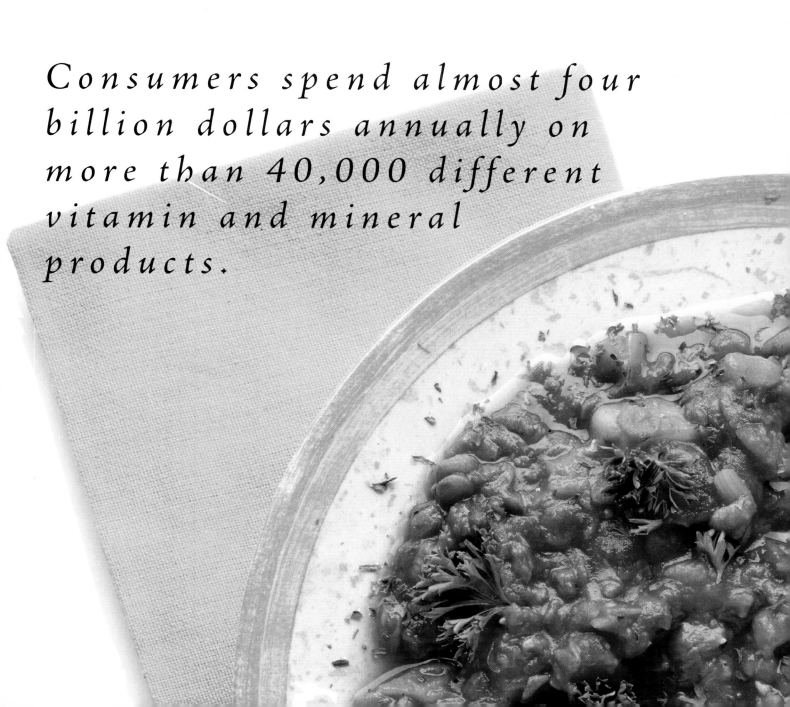

In a large pan mix:

2 cups	Dry lentils
8 cups	Water
1	Medium onion, chopped
½ cup	Celery, diced
2	Cloves garlic, crushed
2 T	Olive oil
2	Bay leaves
¾ tsp.	Oregano
¼ cup	Parsley, chopped

Cook 20 minutes

Then add:

2	Medium potatoes, peeled and cubed
2 cups	Baby carrots, or regular diced carrots

When lentils are soft add:

1 tsp.	Salt, or to taste
1 14-oz.	Can tomatoes, chopped
3 T	Tomato paste

Cook 10 more minutes

✦ **Serves 10**

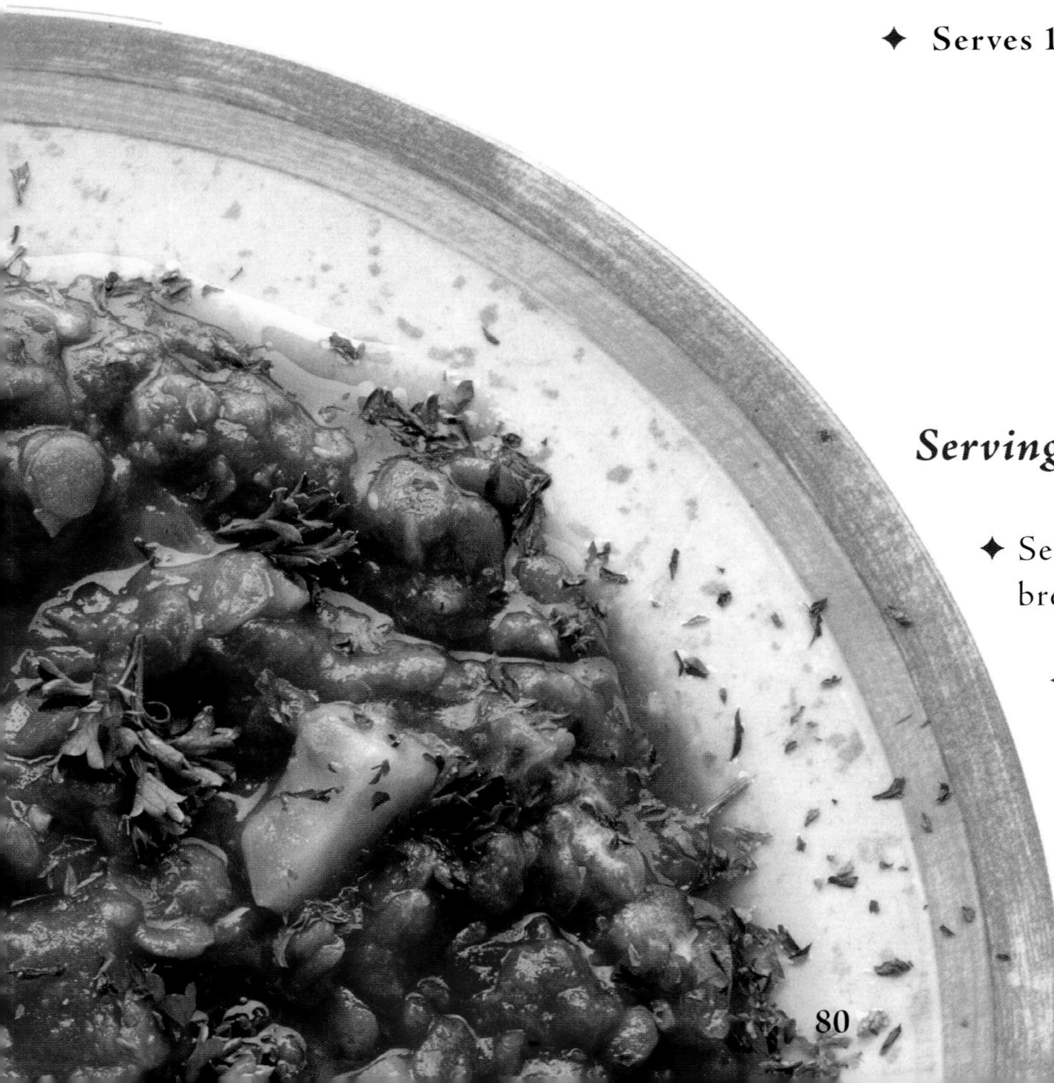

Serving Suggestions

✦ Serve soup with fresh salad and bread.

✦ Serve over a potato, brown rice, or whole wheat toast.

"Many dishes, many diseases. Many medicines, few cures."
~Benjamin Franklin

At this point you may be ready to drop this book and run to the store to load up on supplements. But before you do, please read a little further. Dr. Mary Bielamowicz of the Texas Agricultural Extension Service has this to say:

"Dietary supplementation for the person who is healthy, has food available, and is active is not necessary. Some people may require supplements, but it is not recommended for the general population. Eating a wide variety of foods is the best way to obtain essential nutrients."[64] A regular, consistent, healthy eating pattern is the best defense against irregular, inconsistent, stressful life events!

However, it is true that supplementation may be advisable for certain individuals under certain circumstances. Supplements may be useful for certain inherited metabolic disorders, for premature infants, for women with excessive menstrual bleeding, for peo-

Eating a wide variety of foods is the best way to obtain essential nutrients.

ple with certain injuries, and for those on certain medications. The elderly are often advised to consider increased vitamin B_{12} and vitamin D intake, since the body may lose its ability to absorb these nutrients with aging. Total vegetarians need to

continued on page 90

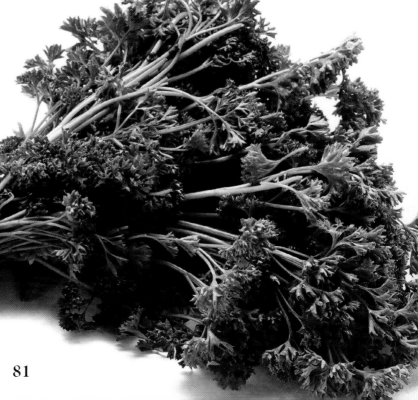

81

More

When you choo...

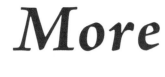

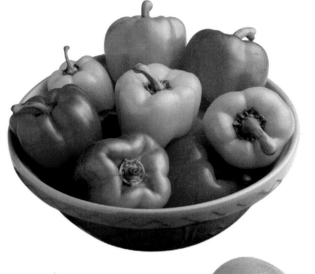

more nutrients:

more quantity:

more fiber and satiety:

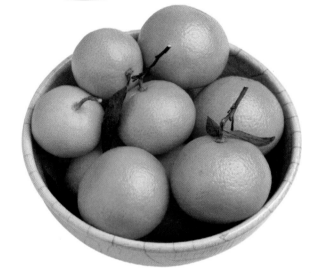

more color:

more flavor:

more variety:

more balance:

more energy:

more productivity:

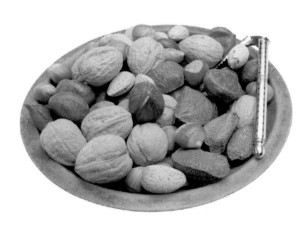

more beauty:

more confidence:

Get More Bounce by the Ounce . . .

Bounce by the Ounce . . . ✦ ✦

od from nature...you get:

    more vitamins, minerals, antioxidants, and phytochemicals;

    more food to eat with fewer calories;

    a fuller and more satisfied feeling;

    beauty on the plate;

    tantalizing tastes from fresh, succulent fruits and crunchy veggies;

    abundance of variety in the produce department;

    a balance of nutrients that are naturally low in calories;

    complex carbohydrates for optimal energy, just ask the athletes;

    a brain that works more efficiently;

    clear skin, bright eyes and slowdown of the aging process;

    to know you are doing the right thing.

You deserve it!

Calorie-Dense

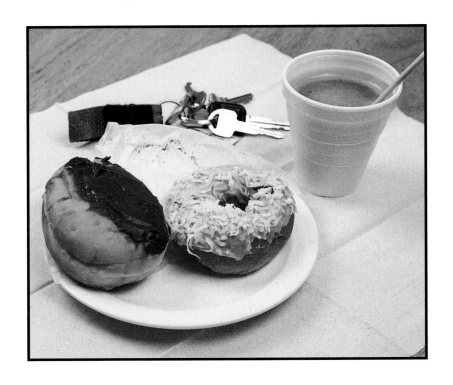

	Calories
2 cream-filled donuts w/icing & nuts	1000
1 cup black coffee	0
Total Calories	*1000*

Calorie-Sense

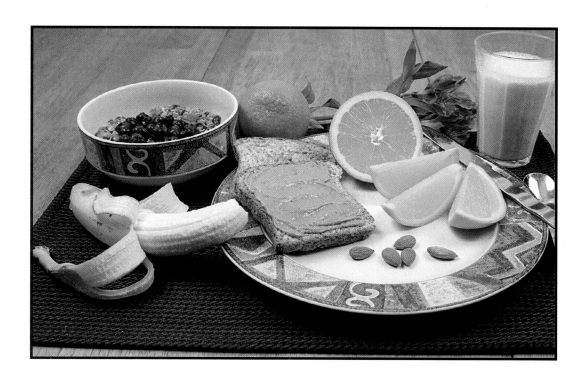

	Calories
5 shelled almonds	40
1 banana	90
1 cup granola	400
2 small oranges	90
1 T peanut butter	100
1 cup soy milk, fortified	130
2 slices whole grain bread, toasted	180
Total Calories	*1030*

Calorie-Dense

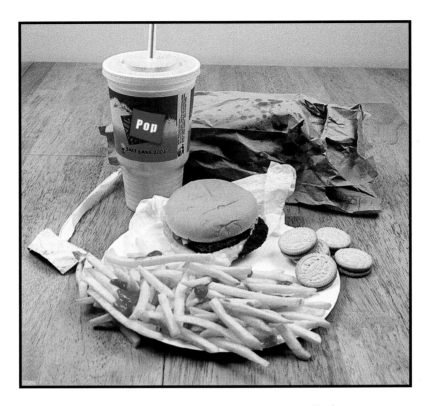

	Calories
1 double burger w/cheese	700
4-oz. cookie	230
l large serving french fries	510
24 oz soda pop	300
Total Calories	*1740*

Calorie-Sense

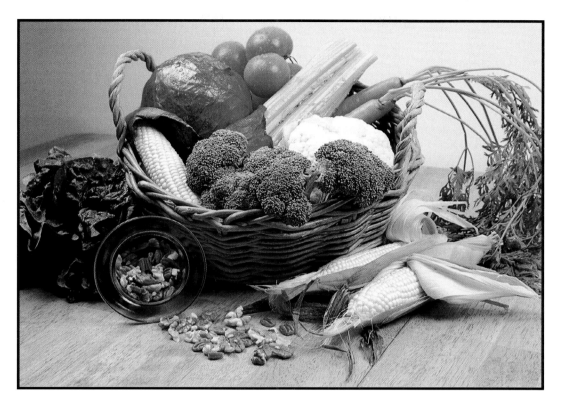

	Calories
1 head broccoli	150
1 head cabbage	100
3 carrots	60
1 head cauliflower	100
1 bunch celery	85
3 ears corn	210
1 head green leaf lettuce	60
1 cup shelled nuts	800
1 head red cabbage	100
3 tomatoes	100
Total Calories	*1765*

Calorie-Dense

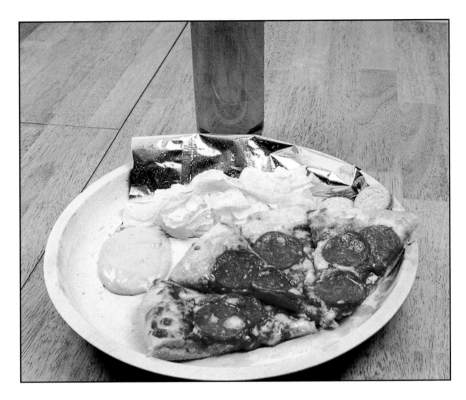

	Calories
3 oz. cheese dip	80
3 oz. chips	390
1 cookie	350
4 slices medium pizza	990
3 cups soda pop	300
Total Calories	*2110*

Calorie-Sense

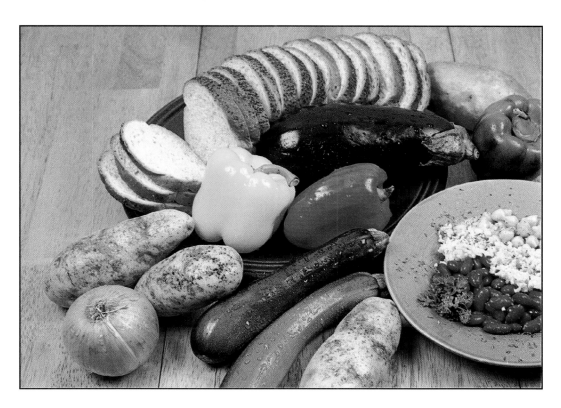

	Calories
½ cup garbanzo beans, cooked	120
½ cup brown rice, cooked	110
1 eggplant	80
½ cup kidney beans, cooked	110
3 bell peppers	45
3 potatoes	300
2 summer squash	100
1 sweet potato	200
1 white onion	50
12 slices whole grain bread	1080
Total Calories	*2195*

Vitamins in the form of pills, liquids, or powdered supplements are no substitute for the real thing.

include a source of vitamin B_{12} in their diet. Supplementation may be helpful during times of extreme stress or chronic pain,[65] although more research is needed. It is always important to check with your doctor regarding supplementation, as supplements can interfere with the action of certain drug medications.

Vitamins in the form of pills, liquids, or powdered supplements are no substitute for the real thing. There are more than 40,000 different vitamin and mineral products available to consumers, who spend almost $4 billion on vitamin and mineral supplements annually.

There is limited evidence indicating the effectiveness of short-term supplementation, while long-term supplementation carries with it several important cautions. It has been stated: "As a principle, adding a relative excess of any nutrient, whether vitamin, amino acid, or intact protein, when others are deficient, may make the situation worse."[66] Trying to correct dietary indiscretions by loading up on supplements could be likened to painting your walls without killing the termites or to plastering paint over a rusty car. Without deal-

90

ing with the underlying problem, you may end up with a worse mess!

Many people reason that if a little of a nutrient is good, then a mega dose must be better! But consistent evidence is lacking. Large, concentrated amounts of one nutrient can interfere with absorption, utilization, or retention of other vital nutrients and have drug-like effects. For example, zinc is essential for the absorption of several vitamins, especially the B-complex vitamins. However, if zinc levels are too high, they disrupt copper use and iron metabolism in the body.[67] If levels are too low, the B complex vitamins are not as effective.

Vitamin E supplementation is very popular, but it poses a similar dilemma. Postmenopausal women who obtained vitamin E from their diet had significant reductions in LDL cholesterol oxidation, which is good news. However, women on vitamin E supplements showed increased LDL oxidation, a damaging effect.[68] Vitamin E is found in numerous forms in foods such as whole grains, green leafy vegetables, nuts, seeds, wheat germ, oats,

Vitamin E is found in numerous forms in foods such as whole grains, green leafy vegetables, nuts, seeds, wheat germ, oats, and unsaturated plant oils.

and unsaturated plant oils. But common sources of vitamin E supplements contain just one, or possibly two, forms—and excessive amounts of one type may displace the kind in the foods that you need! In addition, high doses of vitamin E can cause a decline in vitamin C levels and act as a pro-oxidant, or cell-destroying, agent![69]

People eat vitamin C pills like candy, thinking that because it is a water-soluble vitamin, it must be harmless in any dose. While vitamin C supplementation may be helpful before a bout of exercise to pre-vent exercise-induced asthma,[70] long-term high doses of vitamin C are linked with copper deficiency.[71] Low copper levels are linked to heart disease and osteoporosis. One medium-sized kiwi or an orange meets the daily requirement for this vitamin. Other sources of vitamin C include orange juice, strawberries, grapefruit, mango, pineapple, cantaloupe, broccoli, brussels sprouts, cauliflower, and sweet potato.

Beta-carotene pills have not shown consistent benefits for cancer and heart disease prevention when separated from other food elements[72 73] and may cause harm in smokers and drinkers.[74] Clearly, no nutrient stands alone. There is a complex interdependence that requires balance and caution if the need for supplementation arises.

Supplements can be cost-

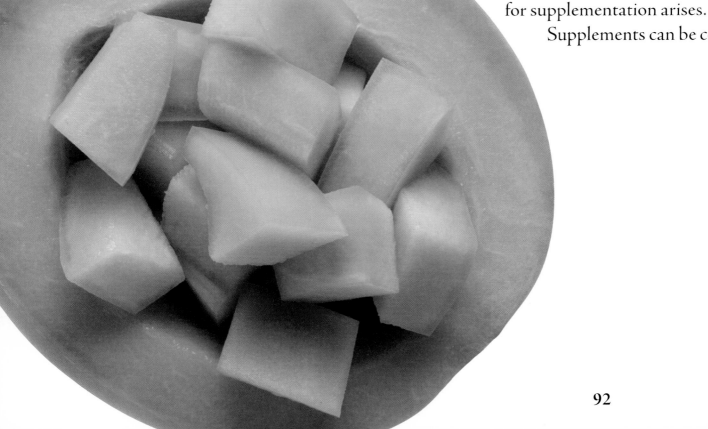

ly, unreliable in their dosing, contaminated, and interfere with other nutrients. To avoid "supplemental trouble," the best first choice is always whole foods!

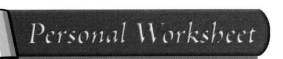

1. What nutritional supplements am I currently taking?

_____

_____

_____

2. What plant sources could I eat to provide these nutrients?

_____

_____

_____

3. What high-sugar, high-fat foods and drinks am I consuming that may be hindering proper assimilation of nutrients?

_____

_____

_____

4. What nutrient-rich foods can I incorporate into my meals that may reduce the need for supplements?

_____

_____

_____

5. Look up Psalm 103:5. What are two promises of God regarding the wholesome foods He has provided? How do they taste?

_____

_____

_____

(see answers on page 123)

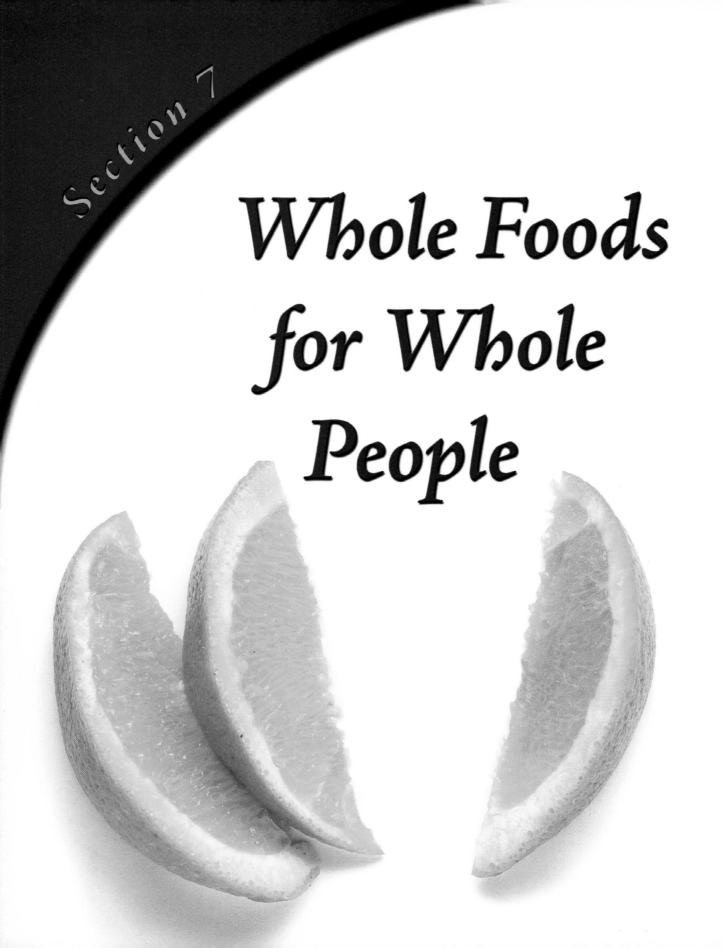

Whole Foods for Whole People

"Whoso diggeth a pit shall fall therein." *Proverbs* 26:27

Haystack Cookies

Mix:

⅔ cup	Peanut butter
⅔ cup	Honey
⅔ cup	Water, cold
1 tsp.	Salt

Add:

⅔ cup	Flour
⅔ cup	Oats, quick
4 cups	Coconut, flaked
1 cup	Nuts, chopped
2 cups	Dates, chopped

Mix together. Using a tablespoon, form balls, pressing each ball together lightly. Place each ball onto sprayed cookie sheet. Bake at 350° for approximately 20 minutes.

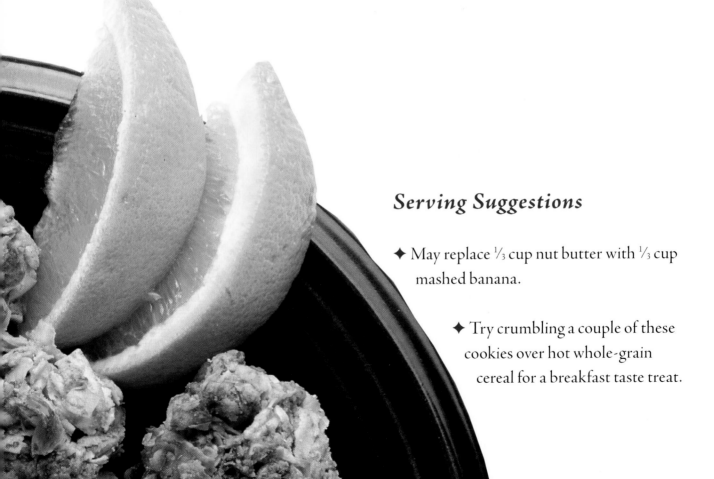

Serving Suggestions

✦ May replace ⅓ cup nut butter with ⅓ cup mashed banana.

✦ Try crumbling a couple of these cookies over hot whole-grain cereal for a breakfast taste treat.

> ## *"The rest of the world lives to eat, while I eat to live."*
> ### *Socrates*

Are you eating your "five a day"? It is recommended that Americans eat at least five fruits and vegetables a day, but most are not. Fresh fruit and vegetable consumption remains unpopular among most Americans, despite the push by the government to increase consumption to five servings a day.

According to a cross-country poll of 5,500 Americans conducted by the U.S. Department of Agriculture, nearly half the people surveyed said they ate no fruit on a given day.[75] Vegetable consumption remains very low, too, with the exception of one vegetable—potatoes. But, unfortunately, the type most chosen is french fries! When people do eat grains, they are often in the form of snack foods such as pretzels, corn chips, and crackers, or lasagna and pizza.

Remember, plant foods and whole grains contain healthful fats, proteins, "complexed" carbohydrates, and macronutrients such as magnesium and vitamins, and many micronutrients and phytochemicals that are essential for proper metabolism, cell protection, and enzyme

> ## *"A person who eats green or yellow vegetables every day shows a lower incidence of stress syndrome (irritation, sleeplessness) than one who does not eat them every day."*
>
> ### *Ann NY Acad Sci 1993;691:281-3*

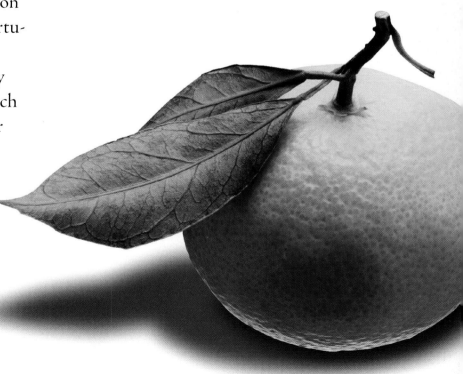

99

and nerve function. When whole plant food consumption goes down, deficiencies go up.

For example, it has been reported that 40 percent of men and about 50 percent of women have inadequate magnesium intake.[76] In addition, numerous studies indicate that either acute or chronic stress can lead to magnesium deficiency.[77] It is interesting to note that a number of the conditions listed earlier that are associated with chronic stress are also linked to low magnesium status.[78] When magnesium levels are less than optimal, the stress response is intensified.[79 80]

Magnesium is a major mineral that is vital for many enzyme systems as well as energy production and muscle and nerve transmission. It is also essential for the proper metabolism of calcium, phosphorus, sodium, potassium, vitamins C and D, and parathyroid hormone. It also may play a

"It is a well established fact that virtually any nutrient deficiency can result in impaired mental function."

vital role in relieving nervous depression.[81] No wonder it is called the "anti-stress" mineral.

People may be tempted to respond to this news by going out and buying magnesium supplements to fill the nutrient gap. But nutrition is a three-legged stool. The right action of nutrients depends on their proper absorption, utilization, and retention. Imbalances of other nutrients can cause a single nutrient to be ineffective or even harmful.[82]

For instance, dietary imbalances such as high intakes of fat and/or calcium can intensify magnesium inadequacy, especially under stress.[83] Laxatives and alcohol also cause the loss of this important anti-stress mineral. Sugar intake has been shown to increase the urinary loss of magnesium and calcium, leading to subsequent alterations in bone metabolism.[84]

But even magnesium does not stand alone when it comes to stress protection or even bone health. Stress levels and bone health are also affected by boron and calcium levels. Green leafy vegetables such as chard, collards, and bok choy are good sources of not only magnesium but also boron and calcium, so they are triple winners! Adequate levels of magnesium and vitamin B_6 have been linked with lower premenstrual syndrome symptoms of anxiety, nervous tension, and mood swings.[85] Again, leafy greens come up winners for B_6 as well as magnesium! Other good plant sources of magnesium include nuts, legumes, whole grain cereals and breads, and soybeans.

Magnesium is just one example of the many nutrients that are delicately balanced within your body to help you maintain good defenses when you are exposed to stress and to lessen the intensity of the stress response when it does occur! And magnesium is an example of the profound effects that low levels of just one of many nutrients can have on the stress system.

It would take volumes to analyze the link between depletion of key nutrients and stress sensitivity, and this is a relatively new field of research. But it has already been noted: "It is a well-established fact that virtually any nutrient deficiency can result in impaired mental function."[86] And according to Melvin Werbach of the UCLA School of Medicine, "It is clear that nutrition can powerfully influence cognition, emotion and behavior. It is also clear that the effects of classical nutritional deficiency diseases upon mental function constitute only a small part of a rapidly expanding list of interfaces between nutrition and the mind."[87]

Plant Power

This new research has also found that plant foods have more power packed in them to protect against stress than just vitamins and minerals. Phytochemicals are an amazing array of compounds that give fruits, vegetables, nuts, and grains their color, flavor, and texture. Some of them even provide stress protection to plants to help them better tolerate heat, cold, drought, and other plant "stressors"! Fruits and vegetables contain 25,000 known phytochemicals such as flavonoids, carotenoids, and terpenoids, some of which have been shown to fight cancer and heart disease; improve memory, learning, and balance, and slow aging.[88]

Phytochemicals have shown an amazing array of health-promoting benefits, as well as offering protection against chronic diseases. If you want to color your life healthy and lower stress levels at the same time, include a wide variety of fruits, vegetables, nuts, legumes, grains, and seeds that include a rainbow of colors: red, green, green-yellow, orange, orange-yellow, purple, brown, and white-green. These colors on your plate beat colored jelly beans every time and are a lot less stressful to your body!

A special benefit of consuming a wide variety of green and yellow vegetables is that they contain hundreds of different types of carotenoids. An interesting study revealed that some of these carotenoids, such as betacarotene, actually have a stress hormone-lowering effect when consumed on a regular basis and are associated with lower levels of irritation and insomnia.[89]

Whole, unrefined fresh foods contain thousands of micronutrients in the right proportions, which is impossible for people to create in the laboratory. God, who created you and knows your body's needs, placed all the right nutrients and compounds in foods, and He placed them in the right proportions for your good. Scientists are still baffled at how slight variations in nutrients such as vitamin E and selenium can significantly alter tissue concentrations and blood levels of these substances! Humans laboring in the laboratory are no match for God the Creator, who created these foods just for you.

You may be saying to yourself, "I know this is right, and I

You may be saying to yourself, "I know this is right, and I need to make changes, but I have no time, energy, or inclination!" Mencius, the Chinese sage, put it this way: "Knowledge imparts information, but not the power to execute." Today it is not so much knowledge that we lack, but power.

Fortunately, the same God who has packed so much power into nature's bounty of foods can also supply stressed human beings with the power to change! "But as many as received him, to them gave he power to become the sons of God, even to them that believe on his [Christ's] name." John 1:12. The same God that is willing to impart His power to do right wants you to reason from cause to effect: "Whoso diggeth a pit shall fall therein." Proverbs 26:27.

Are you in the stress pit? Maybe it's time to climb out!

Are All Calories the Same?

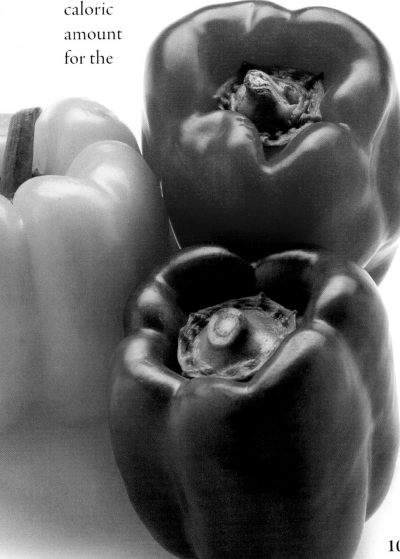

Do you want to lose weight? Or do you want to make sure that you stay at your healthy weight? You know that calories are part of the picture. Does it really matter where your calories come from?

You may have read that one way to lose weight is to count calories. When you reach your caloric amount for the day...you just stop eating. It is true that you will lose weight following this method, but the question is...Can you stay with this method? Do you feel full after a meal and stay satisfied between meals?

An easy way to lose weight is to eat more. Eat more foods with high fill-up value and low in calories. Eat foods that are high in fiber. HIGH FIBER foods fill you up and keep you fuller longer. High fiber foods include fruits, vegetables, whole grains, and beans. When you look at your plate, ask yourself, "Am I eating fiber foods?"

FIBER FOODS are low in calories and high in satisfaction. When you eat a high fiber meal, your appetite will be satisfied until the next meal. You will eat fewer calories. You can reach and maintain your healthy weight. Fiber foods are rich in powerful nutrients that empower your immune system and help you reduce your risk of disease.

Let's look at some groups of foods that contain about 2,000 calories in each group.

Notice the volume of food that you can eat for 2,000 calories when you choose HIGH FIBER foods—foods more like they are found in nature. Notice how concentrated the calories become when they are refined and packed full of fat and sugar. It doesn't take many refined foods to quickly add up to 2,000 calories. How full would you be if you ate 2,000 calories of fruits or vegetables? How long would it take you to eat that much? Could you eat that much? Compare that to how quickly the calories add up if you eat refined foods. It's easy to eat 2,000 calories with fast foods and refined foods. These foods do not satisfy, so you are hungry within a short time.

Reduce your waistline. Go to your produce area and stock up on fresh fruits and vegetables.

Add some whole grains and beans. Get on the right track. Enjoy the delicious variety of colors, textures, and flavors that nature provides.

Sweet Snacks

	Calories
Chocolate bar, 2.13 oz.	260
Apple pie, 4.5 oz.	480
Butter-crunch bar, 2.1 oz.	270
Honey roll, 3.75 oz.	450
Caramel bar, 1.76 oz.	240
Nutty bars, 2.5 oz.	290
Total Calories	*1990*

V◆S

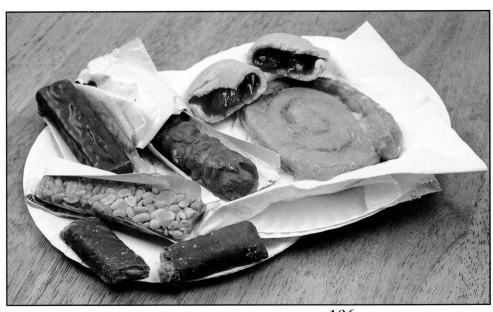

Fresh Fruit

	Calories		Calories
Apples, 2 large	200	Pears, 2 small	200
Bananas, 2	200	Pineapple, 1	155
Cantaloupe, 1/2	80	Walnuts, 1 cup shelled	400
Grapes, 8 cups	400	Watermelon, ⅙ portion	150
Limes, 2	30		
Oranges, 2 small	120	**Total Calories**	**1935**

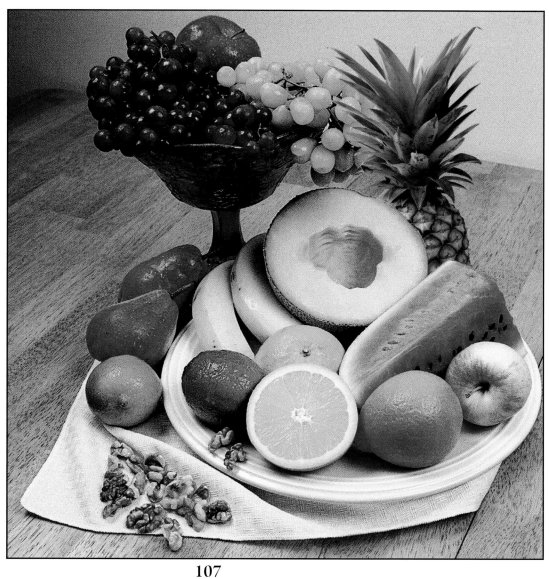

Salty Snacks

	Calories
4 oz. Corn nuts	480
4.5 oz. Corn chips	700
6 oz. Potato chips	780
Regular french fries	340
Total Calories	**2300**

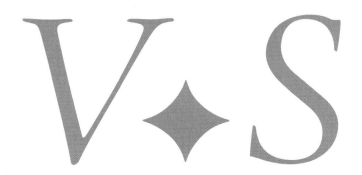

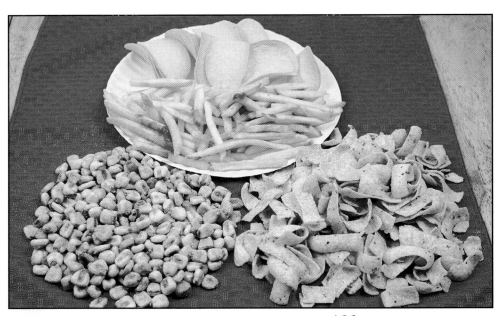

Fresh Vegetables & Grains

	Calories		Calories
Avocado, 1	400	Leaf lettuce, 1 head	60
Cabbage, 1 head	100	Tomatoes, 2	50
Carrots, 3	60	Whole wheat fettuccini,	
Cauliflower, 1 head	100	4 cups cooked	600
Cucumber, 1	30		
Eggplant, 1	80	**Total Calories**	**2225**
Nuts, 1 cup shelled	400		
3 Bell peppers	45		
Potatoes, 3	300		

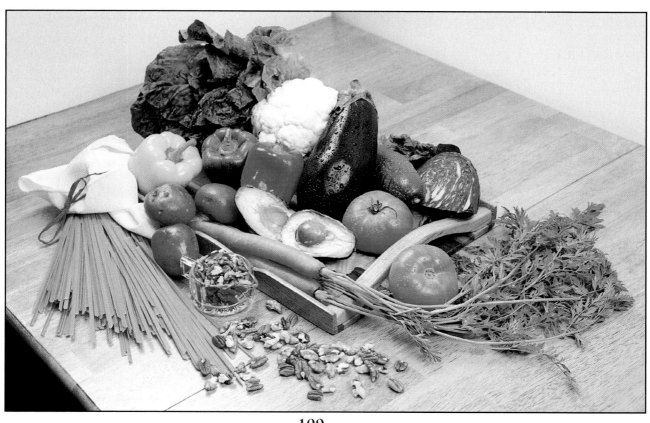

1. Look up Psalm 107:2, 7. What are two promises of God regarding my welfare and happiness?

   _____

   _____

   _____

2. List whole foods (fruits, vegetables, grains, nuts, and seeds) that I really like or am willing to try, according to color groups. Try to include as many in each color category as you can.
   Red: _____
   Orange: _____
   Yellow: _____
   Green/White: _____
   Blue/Purple:_____
   Brown/Black: _____

3. Look up Psalm 107:9 and 3 John 2. What is God interested in besides my physical welfare?

   _____

   _____

   _____

4. Look up Isaiah 63:9. When I suffer, even as a result of my own choices, how does God treat me?

   _____

   _____

   _____

5. Look up Isaiah 27:5 and Deuteronomy 33:25. What help does God offer? How often is it available?

   _____

   _____

   _____

(see answers on page 123)

GLOSSARY

Adrenaline—Also called epinephrine. A hormone that is produced in response to stress, low blood sugar, or other stimuli that causes the release of stored sugar from the liver. It also acts as a stimulant to the sympathetic nervous system, and a neurotransmitter in the central nervous system.

Amino acids—The chemical building blocks of proteins which are synthesized by living cells or are obtained as essential components of the diet.

Anorexia nervosa—A serious eating disorder characterized by an obsessive fear of weight gain leading to faulty eating patterns, malnutrition, over-exercise, and usually excessive weight loss.

Antidepressants—Drugs that stimulate the mood of a depressed patient, including tricyclic antidepressants and monoamine oxidase inhibitors.

Antioxidants—Compounds that prevent or delay deterioration caused by the action of highly reactive forms of oxygen. Antioxidants occur naturally in many foods as nutrients (beta-carotene, vitamin C, E, selenium), or non-nutrients (flavonoids, isoflavones, lycopene).

Atypical depression—Atypical depression is the most common form of depression in outpatients. Symptoms include mood swings, lethargy, and abnormally increased appetite.

Autoimmune disease—Illnesses, which occur when the body tissues are attacked by its own immune system. The immune system is a complex organization within the body that normally seeks and destroys foreign invaders of the body, particularly infections. Patients with these diseases have unusual antibodies in their blood that target their own body tissues.

Beta carotene—A yellow-orange pigment that is converted into vitamin A in the body. The yellow-orange coloring in fruit and vegetables is mainly due to the presence of beta carotene.

Blood sugar—The level of glucose in the blood. Red blood cells and most of the nervous system, including the brain, rely on this fuel to meet most of their energy requirements.

Boron—An essential mineral nutrient found in trace amounts in most tissues. Boron is essential in bone formation in men and women, and may help prevent magnesium and calcium loss in postmenopausal women. Boron plays a role in arthritis and hypertension because of its relationship with calcium.

Calcium—An essential mineral nutrient that is the most abundant in the body. 98% of calcium occurs in the bones and teeth, and constitutes 2% of total body weight. Calcium is also important in nerve transmission, muscle contraction, heart rhythm, hormone production, wound healing, immunity, blood clotting, and blood pressure.

Carbohydrates—A large class of organic compounds that includes sugars, starches, and fiber. Nutritionally important carbohydrates are categorized as simple and complex, according to their size.

Carotenoids—Yellow, orange and red pigments found in yellow and orange fruits and vegetables. They also occur in dark-green leafy vegetables, but the color is masked by chlorophyll. There are more than 500 carotenoids synthesized by plants.

Chromium—A trace mineral element which helps increase the body's sensitivity to insulin in the metabolism of glucose.

Chronic depression—Persistent low-grade depression, also known as dysthymia: Depressed mood is present most of the time for a period of two years, and is accompanied by changes in energy, appetite, or sleep, as well as low self-esteem and feelings of hopelessness.

Chronic excessive exercise—A phenomenon often associated with eating disorders, where exercise is continued in spite of pain or tightness in the chest, irregular heartbeat or rapid pulse that does not decrease after working out, feeling faint or clumsy, or joint pain.

Chronic fatigue syndrome—A persistent condition of prolonged and severe feelings of tiredness or fatigue that is not relieved by rest, and is not directly caused by other conditions.

Cognitive development—The growth of the perceptive faculties, including reason, logic, and mental skills.

Complex carbohydrates—Long-chained sugars that occur in plant-derived foods like fruits, vegetables, and legumes. The two main categories of complex carbohydrates are starches and fiber.

Corticosterone—A steroid hormone that is produced in response to stress that affects protein, fat, and carbohydrate metabolism, and water and mineral balance to a lesser degree. It also possesses anti-inflammatory and immune-suppressive properties.

Cortisol—A major stress hormone that that

affects the metabolism of protein, fat, and blood sugar, and is involved in regulation of stress and immune function.

Cushing's syndrome—An abnormal bodily condition characterized by obesity and muscular weakness due to hyperactivity of the adrenal or pituitary gland, resulting in excessive steroid hormone production.

Dioxin—Dioxin is a general term that describes a group of hundreds of chemicals that are highly persistent in the environment. Dioxin is formed as an unintentional by-product of many industrial processes involving chlorine such as waste incineration, chemical and pesticide manufacturing and pulp and paper bleaching. Dioxin is formed by burning chlorine-based chemical compounds with hydrocarbons. The major source of dioxin in the environment (95%) comes from incinerators burning chlorinated wastes. Dioxin pollution is also affiliated with paper mills, which use chlorine bleaching in their process, and with the production of Polyvinyl Chloride (PVC) plastics.

Dopamine—A hormone and neurotransmitter that is dependent on dietary tyrosine, folic acid, magnesium, and vitamin B12 for synthesis. It is widely distributed in the central nervous system from which epinephrine and norepinephrine are formed. It is a central nervous system neurotransmitter essential to control of motion. Degeneration of certain dopamine-producing brain cells results in parkinsonism.

Dysregulation of the stress-system—Persistent over- or underproduction of stress hormones, resulting in various chronic conditions.

DHA—An abbreviation for docosahexanoic acid, a long-chain omega-3 fatty acid formed from EPA. DHA is preformed in fish oil.

EPA—An abbreviation for eicosapentanoic acid, a long-chain omega-3 fatty acid formed in the body from plant sources of alpha-linolenic acid. EPA is preformed in fish oil.

Flavonoids—A large family of widely distributed plant substances that are often pigments, and are present in especially high numbers in fruits, particularly citrus, purple berries, and apples. They help reduce damage due to inflammation, reduce the risk of various cancers, encourage repair of connective tissue, and help protect the nervous system.

Free fatty acids—Long or short-chain fatty acids in the blood stream that are readily available for the body to use for energy, transport of proteins (lipoproteins) or storage.

Hippocampus—A curved elongated ridge that is a part of the temporal lobe memory system, especially associated with short-term memory, and particularly vulnerable to prolonged stress hormone exposure.

Homeostasis—A state of equilibrium or balance, or a tendency toward such a state between different but interdependent elements or groups of elements.

HPA—An abbreviation for hypothalamus-pituitary-adrenal axis, one of two main branches of the stress system. The major end product of the HPA is cortisol, a stress hormone.

Hydrogenated fats—Vegetable oil that has been modified by the addition of hydrogen. Hydrogenation creates a more saturated fat, and thus hardens or solidifies vegetable oils. Examples of hydrogenated fat include stick margarine and vegetable shortening. Hydrogenated fats are a large source of trans fats, which have documented adverse health effects.

Hyperthyroidism—Overactivity of the thyroid gland due to overproduction of the major thyroid hormone, thyroxine.

Hypothyroidism—A condition resulting from inadequate production of thyroid hormones.

Immune dysfunction—Includes hyper-or hyposensitivity of the body's immune system, either cellular (T-lymphocytes) or humoral (antibodies). Can result in inflammatory conditions, allergy, susceptibility to infection, etc.

Immune system—A complex system of cellular components that help the body distinguish between "self" and "non-self" in the defense against foreign organisms and substances.

Insulin resistance—Insulin resistance is most commonly associated with diabetes. Many people with Type 2, adult onset diabetes produce enough insulin, but their cells do not respond well to the action of the insulin. This is often associated with overweight and high fat diets, and can often be reversed with lifestyle interventions like diet and exercise. Insulin resistance in also linked to elevated blood pressure and high levels of fat in the blood.

Long-chain fatty acids—Long-chain fatty acids are the building blocks of fats and oils and are the major fat components in a typical diet. Long-chain fatty acids may be saturated or unsaturated. Generally speaking, the longer the fatty acid chain, the more liquid the fat at room temperature.

Low—serotonin obesity— Lower than normal levels of serotonin are associated with the control of hunger and appetite. Some obese people have chronically low levels of brain serotonin, which is associated with increased hunger.

Macronutrients—Nutrients required by the diet in amounts ranging from a fraction of a gram to more than a gram. The major minerals calcium, magnesium, sodium, chloride and phosphorus are macronutrients.

Magnesium—A major mineral nutrient. Forty percent is found in tissues like muscle, and 60% occurs in bone and teeth, where it is combined with phosphate. Magnesium is required for major energy producing metabolic processes. More than 300 enzymes are activated by magnesium, and it is essential for the transmission of nerve impulses, muscle contraction, bone density, and maintenance of blood vessels. It has been called a major "anti-stress mineral."

Mercury contamination—Mercury is a toxic heavy metal and environmental pollutant. Once released into the environment, often from industrial waste or combustion of pollutants, it accumulates in the food chain in the form of methylmercury. Because it is fat-soluble, it concentrates in fatty tissues. Predatory fish possess the highest levels. Tuna, shark and swordfish are often contaminated with mercury. Methylmercury acts as a nerve poison, and the brain is especially susceptible to mercury toxicity, especially the developing brain.

Metabolism—The chemical changes in living cells by which energy is provided for vital processes and activities and new material is manufactured and used.

Micronutrients—Nutrients that are required by the body in trace amounts, either milligrams or micrograms. They include vitamins and trace minerals, such as zinc, iron, chromium, copper, iodine, and manganese.

Monounsaturated fats—A type of plant oil that is more healthy than saturated fats. The most common monounsaturates include olive oil, the oil found in avocados, almonds, and nuts, canola oil, and certain sunflower oils. These oils contain comparatively less polyunsaturated fatty acids and saturated fatty acids than other oils.

Motor development—Development that has to do with larger skills in movement, such as muscle coordination.

MUFA—An abbreviation for monounsaturated fatty acid

Nervous-system reactivity—A marked increase in sensitivity to nervous system stimulation, and a strong response when stimulation does occur.

Neuroendocrine—Relating to, or being a hormonal substance that influences the activity of nerves.

Niacin—A member of the B vitamin complex needed by the body to extract energy from fats, carbohydrates, and protein.

Norepinephrine—A chemical neurotransmitter and hormone that is the chemical means of transmission across synapses the sympathetic nervous system and in some parts of the central nervous system. It is a precursor of epinephrine, also called adrenaline, a chemical cousin.

Nutritional deficiency diseases—Diseases caused by inadequate intake of certain vitamins or minerals. Classical deficiency diseases include pellagra, due to niacin deficiency, rickets, which is caused by vitamin D deficiency, and scurvy, caused by vitamin C deficiency.

Obsessive-compulsive disorder—Obsessive-compulsive disorder is an anxiety disorder characterized by the presence of obsessions or compulsions; having one or both is sufficient for the diagnosis. An obsession is a recurrent or persistent thought that is intrusive or inappropriate. A compulsion is a repetitive behavior a person feels driven to perform.

Omega-3 fats—An essential fatty acid. That is, the body cannot manufacture it in sufficient amounts, so dietary sources are important.

Also called alpha linolenic acid, it is the major omega-3 fatty acid, and is a major fat found in plants. Alpha linolenic acid is converted in the body to longer chain omega-3 fatty acids, like eicosapentanoic acid and docosahexanoic acid, which are also found preformed in fish.

Omega-6 fats—An essential fatty acid. That is, the body cannot manufacture it in sufficient amounts, so dietary sources are important. Also called linoleic acid, it is the primary member of the omega-6 family of fatty acids. The body converts linoleic acid to other omega-6 fatty acids, like gamma linolenic acid, dihomogammalinolenic acid, arachidonic acid, and adrenic acid. Vegetable oils and meats are high in omega-6 fatty acids, and overconsumption of omega-6 is associated with numerous chronic and degenerative diseases, like heart disease, stroke, dementia, and arthritis.

Panic disorder—Unpredictable attacks of anxiety that are accompanied by physiological manifestations like sweating, difficulty breathing, and rapid heartbeat.

Partially hydrogenated fats—A vegetable fat that goes through less hydrogenation than a fully hydrogenated fat. Examples of partially hydrogenated fats include most brands of potato chips and corn chips, crackers, tub margarines, frozen pizzas, salad dressing, frozen entrees, baked goods like bread and cookies, and most peanut butters. Partially hydrogenated fats are a large source of trans fats, which have documented adverse health effects.

Phosphorus—A major mineral nutrient found primarily in bones and teeth. It is the most common mineral in the body after calcium, and accounts for nearly 1.5 pounds of an adult's weight.

Physiochemical reactions—Chemical reactions in the body that affect body processes and function.

Phytochemicals—Plant chemicals of a wide variety and type, many of which are known to have health benefits, such as flavonoids, carotenoids, indoles, saponins, and lignans, to name a few. More than 25,000 phytochemicals have been identified, and numerous phytochemicals are thought to protect against cancer and heart disease.

Polychlorinated byphenyls (PCBs)—PCBs are mixtures of synthetic organic chemicals with the same basic chemical structure and similar physical properties ranging from oily liquids to waxy solids. PCBs were used in hundreds of industrial and commercial applications including electrical, heat transfer, and hydraulic equipment; as plasticizers in paints, plastics and rubber products; in pigments, dyes and carbonless copy paper and many other applications. PCBs have been demonstrated to cause a variety of adverse health effects. PCBs have been shown to cause cancer in animals. PCBs have also been shown to cause a number of serious non-cancer health effects in animals, including effects on the immune system, reproductive system, nervous system, and endocrine system.

Polyunsaturated fats—Liquid fats that contain a relatively high percentage of polyunsaturated fatty acids. These are "bent" molecules that contain multiple double bonds, and do not solidify as easily as saturated fats.

Post traumatic stress disorder—Post-traumatic stress disorder is a form of anxiety disorder that is triggered by memories of a traumatic event, either to one's self or others. The disorder commonly affects survivors of traumatic events such as sexual assault, physical assault, war, torture, natural disasters, an automobile accident, an airplane crash, a hostage situation or a death camp. Post-traumatic stress disorder may affect about 1 in 25 adults in the United States. The disorder affects men and women in about the same numbers.

Potassium—A mineral nutrient found mainly within cells. It is a positively charged electrolyte and serves an important role in skeletal muscle contraction, heart muscle contraction, transmission of nerve impulses, and energy release from food.

Premenstrual syndrome—An array of symptoms associated with menstruation, linked to hormone fluctuations, possibly aggravated by poor nutrition. Symptoms can include bloating, discomfort, headache, irritability, insomnia, food cravings, and depression.

Protein loss—Protein and amino acids contain nitrogen, and nitrogen balance is a marker of overall protein sufficiency. Protein loss, or negative nitrogen balance occurs when the amount of protein intake does not compensate for the amount of nitrogen lost. This can occur during starvation, disease, or extreme stress.

Saturated animal fat—Animal fat that contains a high percentage of saturated fatty acids and exists as a solid at room temperature. Saturation refers to the fact that carbon atoms in the fatty acid molecules are bonded to a maximum number of hydrogen atoms. Typical sources of saturated animal fat are beef, veal, lamb, pork, meat products, milk, eggs, cheese, butter, ice cream, and chocolate.

Seasonal depression—Many people, especially women, have described a sense of sadness, loss and lethargy that accompanies the shortened days of fall and winter. Symptoms may also include There are degrees of seriousness of this disorder, and when the depression and lack of energy become debilitating, the condition is called Seasonal Affective Disorder (SAD). It is estimated that SAD affects over 10 million Americans. The milder, "Winter Blues" may affect a larger number of individuals.

Selenium—A trace mineral that functions either alone or as part of enzyme systems. Selenium has antioxidant and anticancer properties, and is thought to be protective against prostate cancer. It is found in highest concentrations in the kidney, heart, spleen and liver.

Serotonin—Serotonin is a chemical messenger found in three major areas of the human body: blood vessels, the central nervous system, and in the intestinal wall. Serotonin is related to mood, appetite, and emotion. Serotonin is involved in the control of mood and the vital functions of the brain. It is essential that the human body has a normal level of serotonin between the nerve cells and in the brain. When serotonin levels are lower than normal, people may suffer from depression or other psychological and physical problems.

Stress response—Refers to the body's physio-chemical reactions to various stres-inducing stimuli, or stressors.

Stress-proneness—The threshold of reactivity to a stressor. A stress-prone individual would have a lower threshold to certain stressful stimuli than a less easily stressed individual.

Stress-sensitivity—See stress-proneness.

Stress-system activity—In this text stress system activity refers to the activity of the hypothalamus-pituitary-adrenal axis (HPA). When a stress response occurs, the hypothalamus produces corticotropin-releasing hormone (CRH), which stimulates the pituitary to produce adrenocorticotropin hormone (ACTHI), which in turn stimulates the adrenals to produce cortisol, a stress hormone. During normal function, through a negative feedback system, the resulting cortisol levels in the brain cause CRH to "turn off" and levels return to normal.

Sympathetic nervous system—A division of the autonomic nervous system that accelerates the heart rate, constricts blood vessels, and raises blood pressure. (The autonomic nervous system regulates the activity of the heart muscle, smooth muscles, and glands.)

Terpenoids—A large family of plant phytochemicals that are lipid-based, including the fat soluble vitamins A, E, and D, and various oils like lemon, orange, peppermint, and ginger oil. Animal terpenoids include cholesterol, steroid hormones, and bile salts.

Thiamin—A water-soluble vitamin and member of the B-complex. Thiamin is essential for the energy production of carbohydrates and fat. The active form also serves as an enzyme helper in the breakdown of glucose. It is essential to the normal function of peripheral nerves, skeletal muscle, and heart muscle, among others.

Tryptophan—A dietary essential amino acid and building block of proteins. Tryptophan is required for the synthesis of serotonin, a neurotransmitter that helps conduct nerve impulses between cells, and is involved in mood, appetite and emotion. Although tryptophan is an amino acid found in protein foods, eating more protein does not increase brain levels. Complex carbohydrates, like breads, pasta, beans, and rice increase the brains uptake of tryptophan and increase serotonin levels.

Type 2 diabetes—Also called adult onset diabetes, or non-insulin-dependent diabetes mellitus (NIDDM). It is a common form of diabetes that develops especially in adults and most often in obese individuals. It is characterized by high blood sugar resulting from impaired insulin utilization (hyperinsulinism) coupled with the body's inability to compensate with increased insulin production.

Tyrosine—A non-essential amino acid that is readily synthesized by the body. Tyrosine is needed for the production of the neurotransmitters dopamine, norepinephrine, and epinephrine. It is widespread in plant and animal foods.

Vascular dementia—Dementia is loss of cognitive and emotional abilities severe enough to interfere with daily functioning and the quality of life. Vascular dementia is dementia that results from insufficient blood flow to the brain, called cerebral insufficiency. Vascular dementia is the second leading cause of dementia, just after Alzheimer's disease.

Vitamin B-complex—The known B-complex vitamins are B1, B2, B3, B5, B6, B12, B15, biotin, choline, folic acid, inositol, and PABA. The grouping of these water-soluble vitamins is based upon their common source distribution, their close relationship in vegetable and animal tissues, and their functional relationships.

Vitamin B12—An essential water-soluble nutrient that is required in minute amounts for cell division and growth, and nervous system integrity. It is the only B vitamin stored in the body. Total vegetarians need to supplement this vitamin.

Vitamin B6—An essential water-soluble nutrient found in two forms, pyridoxine and pyridoxamine. B6 is important for amino acid formation and break down, and for healthy immune and nerve function.

Vitamin C—A water-soluble vitamin that promotes wound healing, healthy blood vessels, joints, gums, and connective tissue. It aids in the synthesis of collagen, a structural protein that provides strength to bones and tissues. An antioxidant, it also occurs in high levels in hormone—secreting glands, and is needed by the adrenal glands to make hormones. It also occurs in high levels in the brain, and plays a role in nerve transmission.

Vitamin D—A fat-soluble trace nutrient that promotes the body's absorption of calcium, which is essential for the normal development of healthy teeth and bones. It also helps maintain adequate blood levels of calcium and phosphorus. It is found in fortified cow's milk and fortified soy, rice, or almond milks, as well as other fortified products like some orange juices and cereals. It is also known as the "sunshine vitamin" because the body manufactures the vitamin after being exposed to sunshine.

Vitamin E—A fat-soluble essential nutrient that stabilizes cell membranes. It comes in several forms naturally, with alpha-tocopherol having the greatest activity in the body. It is a major antioxidant, and plays an important role in immune system health, the nervous system, and the hormonal system.

Vitamin K—A fat-soluble vitamin required for normal blood clotting. It comes in several forms, and is also important in the formation of bone proteins that form the matrix for mineralization and bone-building.

Zinc—An essential trace mineral nutrient required for a wide array of metabolic processes. The highest concentrations occur in the skin, prostate gland, eyes, nails and hair. Over 100 enzymes require zinc for proper function.

ENDNOTES

1 Am Psychol 2000; 55(7):740–749.
2 J Occup Environ Med 1994;36:983–988.
3 Ibid.
4 JAMA 1999; 281(10):942–3.
5 Ibid.
6 JAMA 1992; 267(9):1244–1253.
7 Baldwin, BE. Stress. Journal of Health and Healing. 18(3):54–58.
8 Selye H. The Stress of Life. New York, NY: McGraw-Hill Book Co., 1956.
9 JAMA 1992; 267(9):1244–1253.
10 NEJM 1998; 338(3):171–177
11 Ibid; Trends Endocrin.
12 Met 2001;12:198–203
13 Psychosom Med 2000; 62(5):623–632.
14 Pharm Rev 2000;52(4):595–638.
15 Baillieres Best Pract Res Clin Endocrinol Metab 1999;13(4):583–95.
16 JAMA 1992; 267(9):1244–1253.
17 Ibid.
18 Trends Endocrin Met 2001;12:198–203.
19 J Clin Endocrin Met 1998; 83(6):1842–1845.
20 JAMA 1992;267(9):1244–1253.
21 NEJM 1998; 338(3):171–177.
22 Ibid.
23 Contemp Nutr 1984;9:7.
24 Am J Clin Nutr 1979;32(12 Suppl):2623–2626.
25 Contemp Nutr 1984;9:7.
26 Compr Ther 1985;11(8):21–28.
27 Asterita, M. Physical Exercise, Nutrition and Stress. New York, NY: Praeger Publishers, 1986.
28 Ibid.
29 Stress Medicine 1995; 11(1):1–6.
30 NEJM 1998; 338(3):171–177.
31 Rice, P. Stress and Health, 2nd ed. Moorhead State University. Brooks/Cole Publishing, 1992.
32 Ibid.
33 Nutr Rev Suppl May 1986.
34 Int. J Eating Disord 1996;20(1):105–9.
35 Appetite 1997; 29(3):391.
36 Pediatrics 2000;105(2):E21.
37 J Abnorm Psychol 1985;(94):563–579.
38 The Sciences 1979;7:6–7.
39 Ibid.
40 Rice, P. Stress and Health, 2nd ed. Moorhead State University. Brooks/Cole Publishing, 1992.
41 NEJM 1988;319(7):413–420.
42 Science 1996;273:749–750.
43 J Am Diet Assoc 2000;100(1):43–51.
44 Ibid.
45 WHO report, Jan. 31, 2000.
46 Somer E. Food and Mood. Henry Holt and Company, NY 1995.
47 Ibid.
48 Int J Food Sci 1999;50(6):445–449.
49 Am J Clin Nutr 2000;72(5 Suppl):1410s–1413s).
50 Appetite 1998;31(1):49–65.
51 Int J Obes Relat Metab Disord 1995; 19(11):811–816.
52 Medical Tribune News Service, 1996
53 Exp Aging Res 1997;23:201–235.
54 Mol Cell Endocrinol 1978;12(1):1–8.
55 Am J Physiol 1997;273(6 Pt. 1):E1168–77.
56 Appetite 1997; 29(3):391.
57 Biol Psychiatry 1998; 44(4):243–249.
58 Appetite 1997;29(3):391.
59 Eur J Obstet Gynecol Reprod Biol 1995; 61(1):73–78.
60 J Anim Sci 1998;76(1):142–151.
61 Environ Health Perspect 2001;109(6):605–611.
62 Houlihan J. Brain Food: What Women Should Know About Mercury Contamination in Fish. 2001.
63 Simopoulos A. The Omega Diet. Harper Publishers, NY. 1998.
64 Statement, Texas Agricultural Extension Service, 2000.
65 J Pain Symptom Manage 2000;20(1):1–2.
66 Am J Clin Nutr 1961;9(3).
67 Asterita, M. Physical Exercise, Nutrition and Stress. New York, NY: Praeger Publishers, 1986.
68 J Am Diet Assoc 1997;97(6):655–657.
69 Am J Clin Nutr, March 8, 1997.
70 Arch Pediatr Adolesc Med 1997;151:367–70.
71 J Nutr 1999;129(12):2278–2279.
72 J Natl Cancer Inst 2000;92(12):1014–1016.
73 J Natl Cancer Inst 1999;91(24):2102–2106.
74 J Natl Cancer Inst 1999;91(1):7–9.
75 Medical Tribune 1996 Mar;(Ob/Gyn ed).

76 Exp Gerontol 1993;28(4–5):473–483.
77 Ibid.
78 Magnes Res 1998;11(1):25–42.
79 Artery 1981; 9(3):182–189.
80 J Am Coll Nutr 1994;13(5):429–446.
81 Asterita, M. Physical Exercise, Nutrition and Stress. New York, NY: Praeger Publishers, 1986.
82 Am J Clin Nutr 1961;9(3).
83 Ibid.

84 Bone Miner 1990; 9(3):233–237.
85 J Women's Health Gen Based Med 2000; 9(2):131–9.
86 Am J Nat Med 1995; 2(10):12.
87 Werbach M. Nutritional Influences on Mental Illness; Tarzana, CA: Third Line Press, 1991.
88 J of SC Med Assoc 2000;96:301–303.
89 Ann NY Acad Sci 1993;691:281–283

APPENDICES

High Cost of Stress ...pp. 12–13

[1] Am Psychol 2000: 55:740–749

[2] Am J Psych 2000; 57:360–367

[3] R. Kessler, NCS Comorbidity Study

[4] J Occup Environ Med 1994: 36:983–988

[5] Jama 1999;281:942–3

[6] Surgeon General, May 2001

[7] J Clin Psych 1993;4:425

Social Readjustment Scale ... pp. 14–15

[1] Reprinted by permission of the Journal of Psychosomatic Research, vol. 11, no. 2. pp. 213–218. Thomas H. Holmes and Richard R. Rahe, "The Social Readjustment Rating Scale," Elsevier Science Inc.

Types of Stressors ... pp. 21

[1] Selye, H. Stress Without Distress. New York, NY: Harper and Row, 1974; Chrousos GP. Mechanisms of Physical and Emotional Stress. New York, NY; Plenum Press; 1988.

Altered Nutrition Status

[1] Source: Asterita, Mary F. Ph.D. "Physical Exercise, Nutrition and Stress" Table 10.3, p. 145

Vitamins and Minerals Insert: Sources Asterita M. Physical Exercise, Nutrition, and Stress. Praeger, NY, 1986.

Ronzio R. The Encyclopedia of Nutrition and Good Health. Facts on File, NY 1997.

Craig W. Nutrition & Wellness. Golden Harvest Books, Berrien Springs, MI 1999.

Nedley N. Proof Positive. Nedley, OK 1998.

Melina V. Becoming Vegetarian. Book Publishing, TN 1995.

WORKSHEET ANSWERS

1. Startling Statistics

1. At the end of the world's history, near the time of Christ's second coming.
2. Your answer.
3. Your answer.
4. God has provided spiritual strength, guidance, and lifestyle habits to protect His children from being destroyed by circumstances.
   a. To "put on the Lord Jesus" means to receive Him into a willing heart, and accept his protection, power, guidance, and Divine will.
   b. Avoid any activity or habit, whether mental or physical, that will tend to break down the moral, physical, emotional, or spiritual life.

2. Metabolic Mishaps

1. Your answer.
2. Your answer.
3. a. God promises loving, personal guidance in every area of our lives.
   b. The condition is that we surrender our obstinate wills.
4. a. God's counsel is always true and good.
   b. It is right for all generations, and it is profitable to follow it.
5. a. When we put God's spiritual priorities first, it enables Him to guide us in the daily affairs of life.
   b. God has promised to provide our needs when we acknowledge our need of Him

3. Stress Effects on Nutrition

1. Your answer.
2. Telling the Lord our troubles, exactly as we see them. He will care for us and guide us when there is no one to sympathize or help.
3. Because we reap the consequences of our actions, whether good or bad.
4. Uncontrolled appetite is linked to increased stress and lack of readiness for the second coming of Christ.
5. Physical sickness and spiritual poverty.

4. Nutrition Effects on Stress

1. Your answer.
2. Your answer.
3. Your answer.
4. a. A plant food diet of grains, fruits, nuts, vegetables, and seeds.
   b. They could eat "freely" of these foods.
5. He requested a simple diet of plant foods and water.

5. Fretting About Fat?

1. Your answer.
2. Your answer.
3. a. Because of sin, the earth and its inhabitants are losing vitality and increasing in disease.
   b. God's laws, both moral and physical, have been broken.
4. a. Eating a rich diet with abandon is against God's will.
   b. The result of excess is confusion, moral and physical decay, and temporal loss.
5. Your answer.

6. Plants or Pills?

1. Your answer.
2. Your answer.
3. Your answer.
4. Your answer.
5. a. God will give us satisfying things that have a renewing effect on body, mind, and spirit.
   b. Good!

7. Whole Foods for Whole People

1. God has promised to redeem us from the traps of our spiritual foe, the devil, and He has promised to guide us by the right way in every area of our life.
2. Your answer.
3. God is interested in our spiritual and emotional well-being as well as our physical health.
4. God empathizes with us, pities, us, will redeem us from our past errors, and "carry" us from this day forward.
5. a. God offers us His strength to make changes and go forward.
   b. Strength is promised for each day.

(All references come from the *King James Bible*)

Click Your Way to Better Living!

*I*f you have access to the internet, you have access to some of the best, most up-to-date, scientifically-sound lifestyle resources available. Visit **www.Lifestylematters.com**, produced by the same health professionals who wrote this book. What will you find at **www.Lifestylematters.com**?

✓ *Lifestyle books and videos*
✓ *Up-to-date medical study reports*
✓ *Audio tapes/video tapes/CD's/DVD's*
✓ *Wholesome children's story books*
✓ *Spiritual enrichment resources*
✓ *Online store*

www.Lifestylematters.com
↑ CLICK NOW!

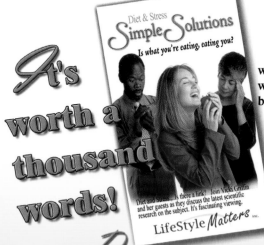

*I*t's worth a thousand words!

*I*f you enjoyed reading this book, you'll love watching to video! It's jammed with information we simply didn't have room to put into the book. What will you see on *Simple Solutions*?

✓ *A lively, informative discussion on the latest studies on stress*
✓ *Tips for reducing shopping stress*
✓ *Stress-cutting lifestyle advice*
✓ *Sometimes humorous, always helpful lifestyle segments*

*D*iet and Stress: Simple Solutions is one of the **LifeStyle Matter**s video series. Join Vicki Griffin, PhD, Edwin Neblett, MD, and Evelyn Kissinger, RD, as they guide you on a fascinating, graphically illustrated journey showing how simple dietary choices can impact stress levels in your life. Order it on our web site. A dynamic power-point presentation on CD is also listed there. Get it, too!

www.LifeStylematters.com

New Toll-Free Number
866-624-5433

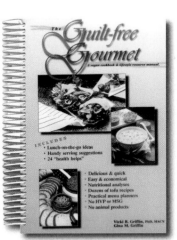

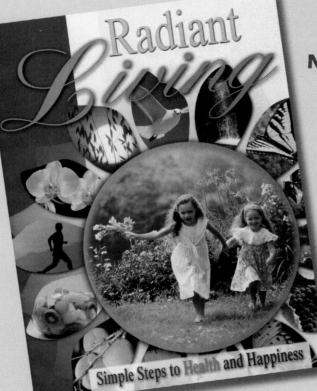

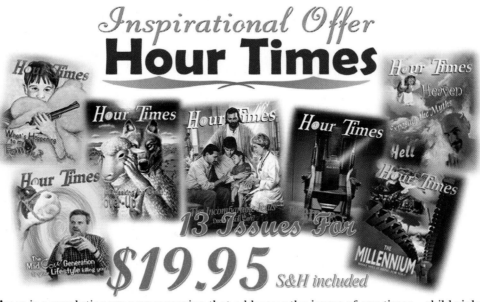

Acknowledgments

The authors gratefully thank the following companies
for donating equipment or materials for this book:

Bed, Bath & Beyond
Belk's Department Store, Asheville NC
Black & Decker Appliances
Calphalon Cookware
Pfaltzgraff Dinnerware
Tupperware
Retinue Dinnerware
Vita Mix Corporation
World Market

Design Staff

COVER:
    Photography: David Sherwin
    Art and design director: Dexter Saddler
LAYOUT:
    Photography: Jason Hanlon and Sarah Spangler
    Layout: Dexter Saddler
    Assistant: Sarah Spangler
ILLUSTRATION:
    Arnold Diaz
EDITORS:
    Sandra Blackmer, Dane Griffin,
    Vicki Griffin,
    Evelyn Kissinger

Pre-production services:

Lithotech, Andrews University
Berrien Springs, MI 49104

Printed by:

IPC Communication Services, Inc.
Saint Joseph, MI 49085

Typeset: Adobe Jenson Pro

PRINTED IN U.S.A.

The information in this book is not intended
to replace medical intervention. Always work with
your physician when making lifestyle changes.

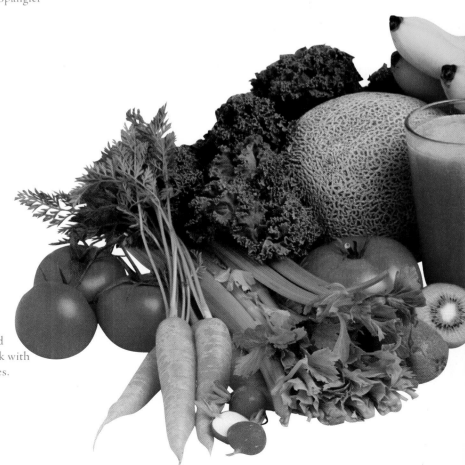

Diet & Stress
Simple Solutions

Is what you're eating, eating you?